"For anyone who has ever been a family therapist or dreamed of being one, Fishman's book brilliantly expands the lens and redirects us to focus on creating coordinated and effective systemic interventions, especially in situations where all systems are failing our children. His book is the clearest, most inspiring and challenging presentation of what it could mean to really deal with human problems from a systemic perspective. It is a breath of fresh air, offering an eye-opening review of our notions of 'evidence' and 'research' and our failure to think and act systemically and effectively in our clinical work. By not paying attention to clients' systemic context or even trying to measure or track the success of our clinical efforts, we have lost our way in misguided non-systemic mental health research and practice. This book can help us turn the corner toward promoting health."

Monica McGoldrick, LCSW, PhD (h.c.), *Director of the Multicultural Family Institute, Highland Park, NJ; Adjunct Clinical Faculty, Rutgers Robert Wood Johnson Medical School*

"*Performance-Based Family Therapy* is a huge leap forward in addressing the woes that limited the growth of system's-based treatment. Fishman has established a clear argument for what is needed to strengthen this field, and it is a model of treatment that is both clearly articulated and provides Performance-Based Accountability. Through his updating of Intensive Structural Therapy and the introduction of outcome measurement tools, this text gives the reader the knowledge and means to practice family therapy in a manner that highlights clinical change and accountability. All therapists, not just those working with couples and families, will benefit from reading his approach and the accompanying case studies."

Scott Browning, PhD, ABPP, *Professor of Psychology, Chestnut Hill College, Philadelphia*

"In this practical clinical guide, Dr. Fishman, a brilliant, early collaborator with Salvador Minuchin and other pioneers in family therapy, stresses the need for a results-based, collaborative family systems approach with struggling youth and families, recognizing larger contextual influences in their distress. His Integrative Structural Family Therapy model, developed for effective training and practice, measures success in light of the strengths and aims of youths and their families, understanding their complex life challenges. His clear guidelines and case illustrations are especially useful for practitioners working multi-stressed families in low-income, marginalized, and under-resourced communities."

Froma Walsh, PhD, *Professor Emerita, University of Chicago;*
Co-Director, Chicago Center for Family Health; Author,
Strengthening Family Resilience, 3e

"Who else, but Charles Fishman, could write a book that brings us closer to understanding the beginnings of family therapy, by incorporating his comradeship with Minuchin, Haley and Montalvo. Inside this noteworthy book, one can see the need for systemic research, the usefulness of Intensive Structural Therapy, and proposals for cost effective treatment, especially children and adolescents, Fishman's forte. Those who have been working in the field will delight in learning the helpfulness of outcome-based supervision as a means of assisting supervisees to develop mastery. Those who are students will have a chance to consider the needs of mental health and where family therapy will fit into our future. This book should be on the shelf of every practicing family therapist and supervisor as a review and assigned as a text for every family therapy student."

Linda Metcalf, *Professor of Graduate Counseling Programs,*
Texas Wesleyan University

"I highly recommend this excellent book. It takes Results Based Accountability (RBA), a framework that has transformed government and non-profit agencies around the world, to the front line of psychiatric care. Dr. Fishman's model integrates Intensive Structural Therapy with RBA and holds the promise for struggling families that therapists will have the capacity to work towards achieving excellent clinical outcomes."
Mark Friedman, *original author of RBA* in Trying Hard Is Not Good Enough: How to Produce Measurable Improvements for Customers and Communities

"In 1981, Charles Fishman co-authored (with Salvador Minuchin) a classic book on family therapy techniques. Now, in *Performance-Based Family Therapy*, he brings us another lucid and highly informative guide to the practice of family therapy."

Michael Nichols, PhD, *Professor, William and Mary College*

"Charles Fishman's latest book not only uncovers the family's hidden strengths, it is also like a reciprocal, juried assessment of our craft – therapists and families alike growing together."

Jay Lappin, MSW, LCSW, *Minuchin Center for the Family*

"Dr. Charles Fishman has dedicated his esteemed career to promoting the benefits of family therapy and advocating for access for economically disadvantaged families. His work is rooted in research into best practices and demonstrating what actually works for family health and well-being. The child welfare field was slow to move away from being primarily child-centered to embracing a whole-family approach, but we finally got it, and Dr. Fishman's work has been instructive. His new book is a brilliant marriage of Results Based Accountability and clinical practice to help the field measure outcomes. It's research, not novelty, and the child welfare field will greatly benefit from this approach. More importantly, it's another tool to help improve family functioning and well-being. Thank you, Dr. Fishman!"

Brenda Donald, *Director, District of Columbia Child and Family Services Agency; Former Deputy Mayor for Health and Human*

"In this most recent book, Dr. Charles Fishman, a renowned clinician and clinical teacher, expands on his previous work in family therapy and presents how the approaches of family systems-based therapy and results-based accountability (RBA) can, in synergy, facilitate the outcome that all clinicians desire the most: measurable change. As summarized by Dr. Fishman, family therapy's '...prioritization of the use of low-cost or no-cost resources was something family therapists intuitively understood in their work. There is no lower-cost resource than the family. A major commonality between family therapy and RBA is that both are in the business of changing systems...'

This very readable and graspable text includes illustrative case vignettes and examples of scorecards, rating scales, and protocols. It promises to be a helpful and practical guide for practitioners and trainees alike. It can further serve to address barriers behind why even the best-conceived treatments do not always translate into meaningful improvements in the real world, where there truly are significant needs for safe, effective, and sustainable mental health interventions for youth and their families. This book describes an integrative, creative, and scientifically grounded method that will likely inspire further approaches to tackling complex challenges in the modern world."

Anthony P. S. Guerrero, MD, Professor and Chair, Department of Psychiatry, The Char, McDermott; Andrade Endowed Professor of Psychiatry, University of Hawai'i John A. Burns School of Medicine

PERFORMANCE-BASED FAMILY THERAPY

In this groundbreaking book, Charles Fishman uniquely incorporates and develops results-based accountability (RBA) into the framework of structural family therapy.

Collaborating with the founder of RBA, Mark Friedman, this approach aims to transform the field of family therapy by allowing clinicians to track performance effectively and efficiently with their clients. The book begins by reviewing the historical foundations of family therapy and evaluates why challenges in the field, alternative methods, and the reliance on evidence-based medicine (EBM) have meant that family therapy may not have flourished to the extent that many of us expected. It then explores how RBA can be integrated into intensive structural therapy (IST), with chapters examining how RBA can be applied in context, such as in treating eating disorders, supervision, and how it can be used to transform the professional's clinical contexts. Relevant and practical, the book also introduces the community resource specialist to help in the treatment of socially disadvantaged families, as well as practical appendices and "tracking tools" to empower clinicians to track their data and choose treatment models that obtain the best outcomes.

This new approach offers transparent and measurable outcomes for both clinicians and training family therapists, lending a helping hand in making family therapy the gold standard in psychotherapy. It is essential reading for undergraduate and graduate students of family therapy, course leaders, and all clinicians in professional contexts, such as social workers, psychotherapists, and marriage, couple, and family therapists.

H. Charles Fishman, MD, a master family therapist, has trained and supervised family therapists all over the world with his primary focus on the "power of the family." He has co-authored with Salvador Minuchin a foundational text in family therapy and five other books, including *Enduring Change in Eating Disorders: Interventions with Long-Term Results* (Routledge).

PERFORMANCE-BASED FAMILY THERAPY

A Therapist's Guide to Measurable Change

H. Charles Fishman, MD

Routledge
Taylor & Francis Group

NEW YORK AND LONDON

Cover image: © Getty Images

First published 2022
by Routledge
605 Third Avenue, New York, NY 10158

and by Routledge
4 Park Square, Milton Park, Abingdon, Oxon, OX14 4RN

Routledge is an imprint of the Taylor & Francis Group, an informa business

© 2022 H. Charles Fishman

The right of H. Charles Fishman to be identified as author of this work
has been asserted in accordance with sections 77 and 78 of the Copyright,
Designs and Patents Act 1988.

Library of Congress Cataloging-in-Publication Data
A catalog record for this title has been requested

ISBN: 9780367746698 (hbk)
ISBN: 9780367751616 (pbk)
ISBN: 9781003161257 (ebk)

DOI: 10.4324/9781003161257

Typeset in Joanna
by Deanta Global Publishing Services, Chennai, India

To Tana, with love

CONTENTS

PREFACE

For therapists whose life's work is helping others sort out their uncertainties, wouldn't a clear, research-grounded healing and practical path forward be useful? Yes, it would. And it's here. Welcome to the second evolution!

Years ago, there was a transformative shift in mental health. Systems thinking and family therapy taught us that "I" of the individual is inescapable from the "we" of context. It was as if therapists were given a new map that included the family within the longitude and latitude of its' social and cultural contexts—a path that didn't just "fix" the patient alone, but rather tapped the entire family system whose underutilized strengths were hidden by the underbrush of sameness.

Charles Fishman's latest book not only uncovers the family's hidden strengths, it is also like a reciprocal, juried assessment of our craft—therapists and families alike, measurably growing together.

Results-based accountability therapy is the means toward that transformative end, for families, larger systems, and for the therapists whose life's work it is to heal those whom we are privileged to serve. Treat yourself to a bite of the apple and Welcome to the Evolution!

Jay Lappin, M.S.W., LCSW,
Minuchin Center for the Family

ACKNOWLEDGMENTS

On a blustery South Pacific Monday morning, I called Mark Friedman, the developer of results-based accountability (RBA). I was asking for help. I was in a new position to clinically direct a national program for out-of-control youngsters. The communities of New Zealand had had enough of the midnight chases in stolen cars. We needed a solid framework to track outcomes and demonstrate that what we were doing was making a difference.

I was confident that RBA was uniquely well-suited for this challenge. When I described the imperative to Mark, he was open to the idea and looked forward to collaborating. RBA had been developed for vast government populations and here I was asking Mark to retrofit his system for front-line care.

In my new country, on the other side of the world, so far away that it was already tomorrow, our work together began. We integrated intensive structural therapy with RBA and rallied all of the stakeholders with a common mission: come together, plan care, intervene, and measure. Thank you to Mark Friedman, the RBA genius, who was willing to step into a different domain and find synergies; you were always available.

I am grateful and fortunate for the generous assistance I received, not only from Mark, but from so many, in the crafting of this book.

A special thank you to Suzanne Faigan, PhD, who, with ever good cheer, expertly helped and supported bringing this manuscript to fruition. Her tireless commitment, along with her excellent organizational skills, were instrumental in achieving this final manuscript.

Jay Lappin, MSW, my dear friend and colleague since my Philadelphia Child Guidance Clinic days, has been, as always, encouraging and an incisive sounding board. My friends Scott Browning, PhD, and Froma Walsh, PhD, offered wise counsel and comradery. Trisa Danz, MD, my child psychiatry colleague, provided razor-sharp feedback. Whaea Rahera contributed cultural tikanga (the customary system of values and practices), making us wiser. Thank you all.

I want to acknowledge the Fellowship Program of the Annie E. Casey Foundation, where I met Mark. The Fellowship is a brilliant executive leadership platform. It has helped to improve the life circumstances and prospects of children and families living in low-income communities these last 30 years. My Casey Fellow colleagues have greatly enhanced my understanding of the inequities of disenfranchised populations.

I have special gratitude for Heather Evans, my editor at Routledge, for her immediate understanding and appreciation of RBA and its value to this book for advancing the field. Her kind, expert validation has been important. Also at Routledge, Upasruti Biswas, for her clear messaging and timely administrative support.

My dear wife of many decades, Dr. Tana Fishman, receives my undying appreciation, not only for her endless support, but for the many hours she and I spent editing these pages. Editor extraordinaire, Tana word-smithed my lumpy prose. Thank you.

And our loving children and grandchildren, I thank you for being the Mensches that you are!

Disclaimer: Information contained in this book accurately conveys the spirit of my work as a family therapist; but all names, characteristics, identifying details, and clinical data of the case histories have been changed.

INTRODUCTION

I was treating Bonnie, a hollow-eyed 16-year-old with severe anorexia nervosa, many decades ago; the treatment I was providing sealed my commitment to family therapy. She ate her lunch during the therapy session; an almost instantaneous response to an intervention. These starving children would often eat within the first or second therapy session—convincing me and others that family therapy is the most effective clinical intervention. A simple "lunch session," where the parents are united to supervise or even feed their child, transforms the family system, while the emaciated, anorectic child starts to eat.

In the 1970s, children with anorexia would be hospitalized for weeks, and sometimes months. They were usually fed by a nasogastric tube and underwent some rudimentary behavioral interventions. Such suffering, where an incorrect form of treatment prolongs the clinical problem, was unnecessary. Yet, even today, many years later, long-term inpatient treatment continues.

All of us at the Philadelphia Child Guidance Clinic (PCGC) were convinced that family therapy and its extraordinary effectiveness was the treatment of the future. Sadly, time has proven us wrong; it was not to be. Disappointingly, family therapy appears to be marginalized. Today, the most utilized psychotherapy is cognitive behavioral therapy (CBT), a type of individual psychotherapy in which negative patterns of thought

DOI: 10.4324/9781003161257-1

about the self and the world are challenged in order to alter unwanted behavioral patterns.

This book is about what went wrong with family therapy and what we, as professionals in this field, can do to expand our much-loved paradigm.

My Early Introduction

I have used this potent model in treating many families over the years. Upon reflection, family therapy principles made sense to me even at a young age. Children learn from their families; if their parents are farmers, they learn how to milk cows and look after livestock. In families that are involved with stores, the children learn the retail world early on.

Ironically, I think the groundwork for the "family business" for me as a future family therapist was in my very early years with my mother, who was forced to leave college to support her immigrant family and spent many decades as a volunteer social worker. Often, we would read a column together in the Ladies' Home Journal called "Can This Marriage Be Saved?" We would discuss the cases and make pronouncements. I don't recall if the column informed readers about the success of its expert's suggestions. I suspect that, like most of the psychoanalytically influenced world at that time, no one was tracking outcomes.

I did some vicarious "field work" when I was about eight years old. One evening, my aunt and uncle came over, distraught, seeking advice from my father. Their 16-year-old son was pressuring them to sign the documents permitting him to quit high school. To make matters worse, he was imploring them to buy him a cheap car—a "jalopy." My father, an eminently sensible lawyer, warned against both. I can still hear him saying, "These are terrible ideas, you're rewarding him for failure." In the next week, his parents, probably quite divided, bought him the car as he walked away from his education. I saw my cousin struggle vocationally after that fateful decision—going from job to job, never able to fully support himself.

Even at my tender age, my father's advice made perfect sense to me. My aunt and uncle were failing their son, or so I must have heard my education-loving parents say. My parents greatly appreciated the parental role in a child's academic success. I saw first-hand how influential parental decisions are in the trajectory of a child's life.

I came of age in the 1960s; our generation was socially engaged and pushing back against the Vietnam War. There were so many radical ideas poised to change the world: civil rights, women's liberation, and the sexual revolution. Attending Lake Forest College and the University of Chicago, majoring in philosophy, I was looking for answers for the worldwide societal turmoil. Disenchantment was washing over me; too many philosophical schools of thought began to appear like so many competing religions. Nobody changed anybody's mind during their interminable verbal wrangling. I struggled with a plethora of elaborate theories—exciting, at times, and compelling—but there was no data to judge the veracity of one model over another. In my philosophy studies, only one theory interested me: pragmatism, which posited, "If it works, it's true." I was liberated upon graduation from the data-free zone of philosophy; it was my great escape.

I boldly marched into the field of science two months after obtaining my undergraduate degree. The study of medicine, at the Medical College of Wisconsin, offered my much-needed respite. I found a genuinely scientific methodology for vetting theories. For example, working in the hospital, if a patient was failing, we would adjust their medications. The next morning, examining their blood test results, we could determine whether the change in medications was making the desired difference. However, in spite of the beautiful, scientific foundation of internal medicine, I was drawn to psychiatry, where the mysterious diseases of the mind were unmeasured and offered opportunities for exploration.

At 25 years of age, I had completed university and medical school. Making a decision that could impact the rest of my life was now my reality. Choosing to train in psychiatry, I was adrift with the panoply of schools of thought within the discipline. I chose the University of Pennsylvania School of Medicine, which offered a rich, broad-based program that could shape my future direction. There were robust departments of psychopharmacology and addiction medicine. In Philadelphia, at the time, there were even two psychoanalytic institutes, actively recruiting. Moreover, family therapy was in its naissance and gaining in popularity. Luminaries, such as Aaron Beck, developer of CBT, and Salvador Minuchin, were teaching within the department.

In those days, psychoanalysis was most influential in the field of psychiatry. The majority of the psychiatrists and psychologists teaching on the faculty were psychoanalysts. Again, I was back to the "Tower of Babel," sitting in philosophy class becoming bored and irritated. There was theory but no grounded data. And with Beck's CBT, I began to doubt the value of those subjective questionnaires. My psychiatric training continued with some disillusionment and a few notable points of interest.

The seminars with Ivan Nagy, the founder of contextual family therapy, created optimism with his theory of change focused on the patient's indebtedness to their family of origin. From his consultations, one anecdote that stands out in my memory was about a psychotic young woman. After he conducted an initial family therapy intervention, her psychotic symptomatology exacerbated; after the second intervention, her symptoms abated. Perhaps the increased expressed emotion in the family played a part, but I thought, "I have no idea of the mechanisms, but this is powerful."

Another sentinel experience for this future family therapist occurred shortly after I began my medical internship. With surprise and terror, I was put in charge of a psychiatric unit over a holiday weekend; a mammoth, block-long, municipal hospital, Philadelphia General. Around midnight, the head nurse urgently alerted me that a young man, whom they referred to as "Big Herb," had been admitted; a mountain of a man, he was six foot five and floridly psychotic. The nurses informed me that during his previous admission, they were forced to call the police, who had tackled Herb to the floor as the nurses sedated him. With trepidation, I entered the unit. I saw "Big Herb" in the nurses' station toying with the earrings of a young nurse. I quickly called my chief resident, a seasoned psychiatrist who had served in the military. Calmly, he told me, "These guys often have wiry little mothers who can easily control them." Surprised and desperate, I called his mother, imploring her assistance. Entering the unit, she walked up to Herb, who physically dwarfed her, took him by the hand, looked him in the eye, and said, "Herb, what are you doing?" She sat him down on his bed, telling him to control himself. The crisis was averted. Her entrance was an enduring lesson for me in the sheer power of families.

Despite these scattered high points, by the end of that second year of general psychiatry training, I was becoming increasingly disheartened. I wondered, "Am I not getting it?" or was there just so little there? My colleagues seemed to be happily in step with the program and that unnerved me even more. I would attend conferences and hear ponderous words like *overdetermined*.[1] Whew. There I was, swimming in theoretical assumptions with little empirical data supporting the models of psychotherapy; just postulates.

The Philadelphia Child Guidance Clinic

During this period, I would hear rumors that across campus at the Philadelphia Child Guidance Clinic (PCGC), Minuchin and his colleagues were curing diabetes with family therapy. (Of course, they were not curing the physiological disease; the family therapy team was decreasing the family stress that caused the diabetic symptomatology to exacerbate.)

In those days, PCGC was to family therapy what Paris was to the art world in the 1920s—a great hub of innovation. People came from all over the world to be trained. Located within the beautiful, brand new, Children's Hospital of Philadelphia (CHOP), the clinic was purpose-built to facilitate working with families. It even had two family apartments with one-way mirrors in the living rooms, where family interactional patterns could be observed and studied. There, the family was truly the "patient." There were professional videographers to record therapy sessions, with a large library of classic tapes.

PCGC was home to some of the early titans of family therapy, who were establishing the foundations of the paradigm, often in heated discussions. Among these great disputants were Salvador Minuchin, Jay Haley, and Braulio Montalvo.

By serendipity, I found myself with a unique opportunity to shift my direction of training and start a child psychiatry fellowship program.

---

1 Overdetermined—the phenomenon whereby a single observed effect is determined by multiple causes, any one of which might be sufficient in isolation. In the case of dreams, Freud observed that they were overdetermined in that they were in one sense informed by proximate events (e.g., an experience had during the previous day), events further in the past, existing template ideas about people, etc.

The evening before the fellowship was to begin, I bumped into a fellow psychiatric resident. "Charles," he said, "I'm not going to the PCGC for child psychiatry. Carol just had a baby. I'm going into private practice." This coveted position was now available! I leaped at the opportunity and met with Dr. Minuchin the next morning.

At this point, Dr. Minuchin had turned his back on psychoanalysis, calling it "a waste of time" and was now an emerging leader in the revolutionary family therapy movement. He extolled the virtues of working with the family, transforming the contemporary system. I questioned him whether this was "deep therapy." At the time, the psychoanalytic culture had splashed over me. The belief of my teachers was to delve into the unconscious and plumb the depths of the patient's psyche. His response was quick: "With family therapy, you change all the members of the family and they jointly support each other in maintaining the changes of the new system." We had a long meeting, and finally, somebody made sense! As he described his ideas, my understanding of clinical work began to change, going from black and white to color—more detail and greater depth. So began my years at PCGC.

The Titans: Haley, Minuchin, and Montalvo

The ground-breaking book, Families of the Slums, published in 1967, by Salvador Minuchin, Braulio Montalvo, Bernice Rosman, Bernard Guerney, and Florence Schumer, was extraordinary (Minuchin et al., 1967). Many decades ahead of their time, the authors delved beyond the troubled child to his or her family context. In one of my last visits to the then aged master clinician, I asked Dr. Minuchin how he had arrived at such an innovative idea. He said:

> My secretary was a brilliant woman. One day when typing my Wiltwyck admission assessments, she said, "You know, Dr. Minuchin, you dictated the same thing about this boy when he was admitted here last year. I thought, "Something is missing in the treatment; maybe we should look beyond these boys and include their families in the treatments."

> (Personal communication, 2021)

Jay Haley

My first supervisor at PCGC, Jay Haley, founder of the strategic model of family therapy, was, as luck would have it, my neighbor in University City in West Philadelphia. We would often walk to and from the clinic together; the conversation was so vigorous and fresh, the previous training, "groupthink", began to recede. Jay was known to be a visionary and a rebel. On our walks, he challenged much of what my non-family therapist teachers were propounding; he dismissed psychoanalysis. One day, fresh with these thoughts, I met with another of my required fellowship supervisors, a senior psychoanalyst. Rushing into his office, I pronounced, "I no longer believe in the unconscious." This middle-aged, elegantly suited analyst, his hand slightly shaking as he juggled his coffee, paused. I can still see his reddening face, desperately trying not to spill the contents of his mug onto his antique oriental rug. This was not what someone from the prestigious Institute of Pennsylvania Hospital wanted to hear.

Jay, as a young man, had worked closely with Gregory Bateson, the biologist and anthropologist, whose writings provided some of the theoretical basis of family therapy. Bateson's concept, *mind in context*, recognized that contemporary social forces were dominantly influential to psychological problems; this concept has remained central to my work.

Jay collaborated with Don Jackson, another of the founders of family therapy. Jackson, a psychiatrist, introduced the fundamental concept of family homeostasis to our field. This concept has enlarged my structural family therapy model to intensive structural therapy (IST), using the assessment lens of the homeostatic maintainer (HM).

In one of Jay's controversial publications, *The Power Tactics of Jesus Christ* (Haley, 1969), he took on the no less redoubtable institution of Christianity, expounding the premise that Jesus was a shrewd leader who understood systems, manifesting his rebelliousness. In many other writings, he again challenged the prevailing orthodoxies of psychology and psychiatry.

Jay embodied the political courage and social commitment consistent with the culture of the Philadelphia Child Guidance Clinic. Jay and Braulio Montalvo spearheaded the development of a program in inner-city

Philadelphia, a branch of PCGC, called the Institute for Family Therapy (IFT). They selected people from this community, people with vast life experience without formal university study, and trained them to be family therapists. Their contrarian position was that life experiences and common sense were more important than academic degrees—life was a great teacher, especially about families. Many of these people proved to be excellent family therapists, and I held onto this daring insight.

Jay supervised a number of my cases. His innovative thinking was at the outer margins of conventional psychiatric theory. Schizophrenic symptomatology, according to Jay, exacerbated when parents triangulated their child. For example, Jay supervised my treatment of a 21-year-old young man with a diagnosis of schizophrenia. At that early point in my training, I was looking for documentation that the "systems model" was more valid than the individual paradigm. As Jay and I worked with this family, I was increasingly struck by the dynamics between the parents. The levels of psychosis of the young man waxed and waned in relationship to the parents.

Salvador Minuchin

My second supervisor at PCGC was Salvador Minuchin. He was born in a small town in Argentina; I believe his father had a grocery store. After medical school, he went to Israel, where he was a doctor in the country's War of Independence. By his own self-description, "I was a wandering Jew" (personal communication, 1982). He left Israel for New York, where he directed the Wiltwyck School for Boys. He had trained as a child psychiatrist and psychoanalyst, and also studied anthropology. Sal had an incisive brilliance and a fierce social conscience. Throughout his 96 years, he fought for the underdog.

He was a great scientific thinker. His contribution of "family structure" provided the clinician the ability to observe grounded data in order to assess the family system and readily track clinical progress.

Braulio Montalvo

My third and most enduring teacher, Braulio Montalvo, was my closest friend for 40 years until his death. Braulio grew up in a tiny town in

Puerto Rico and was trained as a psychologist at Columbia University in NYC. He was a brilliant conceptualizer, therapist, and supervisor. While still a young man, he entered the field by joining Minuchin at the Wiltwyck School for Boys in New York. Together, they developed a model of successfully treating the impoverished families from Harlem. This work was immortalized by their publication, Families of the Slums (Minuchin et al., 1967). Braulio was a viruoso analyst of family process; his edited and narrated videotapes significantly advanced this modality of family therapy training. "The Professor," as I called him, influenced my clinical skills; he gave me a lens to understand the primacy of contemporary family systemic interactions. Salvador Minuchin, in his book Families and Family Therapy (1974), described Braulio as a person to whom you could give an idea and he would give it back to you, greatly enlarged (p. vii). He was a great support and inspiration to me, providing indispensable critiques of my writing. A cherished and loving comrade.

By the mid-1990s, I had been a family therapist for some 20 years. My outcomes seemed to be excellent but what I questioned was the endurance of these changes. I began to wonder whether this transformation of the contemporary system, and the resolution of their symptoms, was maintained over time. With some trepidation, I decided to attempt a clinical audit with families whom I had treated five to 20 years previously. A few I could not locate, but those that I did were happy to discuss their earlier treatment. One of the patients had struggled with severe anorexia beginning two decades before our therapy. She gorged one to two boxes of laxatives daily, often resulting in an electrolyte imbalance requiring medical hospitalizations. Nineteen years had passed since her treatment with me. When I spoke to her husband, he said that Dorothy, sadly, was very unwell with cancer. He went on to say that her anorexia never recurred after our work together.

My findings of this audit were published in my book Enduring Change in Eating Disorders: Interventions with Long-Term Results (Fishman, 2004). The sustainability of these clinical changes in the microsystem inspired me to consider the use of these systemic concepts in the larger public arena. Back to my 1960s optimism and the idea that you could tackle old-fashioned, lumbering, bureaucratic systems. If we could use family therapy techniques to change how a health care system work and how care is delivered, then perhaps we could help even more children and families.

When I mentioned to Braulio that I was considering making a change to working in public systems, he informed me that he had nominated me for the Annie E. Casey Foundation's fellowship program. This was a unique opportunity to work along side leaders in the field of service to children. After an interview and the completion of a competitive process, I was selected.

The Annie E. Casey Foundation, based in Baltimore, Maryland, is funded by United Parcel Service (UPS), established in 1907. The Foundation's webpage describes their focus: "devoted to developing a brighter future for millions of children at risk of poor educational, economic, social, and health outcomes" (The Annie E. Casey Foundation, n.d.). The fellowship focused on improving the leadership of services provided to economically disadvantaged children and their families. During my year-long position, I reviewed treatment programs in several states that were deemed to be "best practices" for treating troubled youth. These programs for economically distressed multi-problem families embraced the "wraparound model." All services, family and community, worked together on a stabilization plan tailored specifically to each child and their family. Ample resources were provided, but the family systems were often not transformed. There appeared to be a scotoma—a blind spot—for the fundamental conflicts of the family, usually within the parental dyad. I am not suggesting that they did not provide family therapy but, if they did, it did not appear that they addressed that component that would lead to sustainable change. The program's focus was not on the warring microsystem but rather more administrative—ensuring that all the boxes were checked.

When the fellowship was completed, I returned to Philadelphia and accepted the position of Chief Medical Officer of a new Medicaid Behavioral Health Maintenance Organization (HMO). This newly formed non-profit corporation, a subsidiary of the city's health department, was innovative; the city itself was providing these services rather than contracting services from for-profit HMOs, the customary practice at the time. This community-based organization worked closely with recovered adult consumers and provided support and advocacy for unwell psychiatric patients. In the children's domain, a family network was organized by the team for struggling families.

One of my major responsibilities was to access and authorize treatment for troubled children and adolescents in this vast system. There were 500,000 covered lives, all desperately low-income families. The most daunting part of the job was finding the programs with the best outcomes. Instead, unfortunately, it became a capacity-based referral process, who had time. The programs/therapists did not systematically track their outcomes, and on that basis, it was difficult to determine whether their treatment was effective.

There was more than adequate medication treatment, wraparound services, and ubiquitous CBT, but a paucity of family therapy, which would likely have transformed these struggling young people's problems. Witnessing this scarcity of service reinforced to me that family therapy was working at the margins. On reflection, it was surprising that this treatment was not available everywhere, especially in Philadelphia, where some of the major models originated. That was not the case. CBT and psychotropic medications were the order of the day.

After three years working in this huge system, I found myself yearning to develop a front-line family therapy program that would more effectively address the needs of young people and their families and provide a clear outcome-tracking system as a model that would serve to instruct HMOs or other purchasers of services. A transparent approach, cost-effective and where everyone is better off.

The funding doors in Philly were closed and a most surprising offer, from the other side of the planet, where the seasons are opposite, and so far away that today is "already tomorrow," was very attractive. The opportunity to develop one such initiative in Auckland, New Zealand, was in front of me.

Auckland, New Zealand

We departed Philadelphia on December 24 and landed in New Zealand, early in the morning, on December 26 (Boxing Day), and the beginning of summer. The 25th of December was lost somewhere over the dateline. Midday, we ambled to the only restaurant we could find open for lunch.

My wife ordered, "Hot tea, please." The waiter stated with certainty that that was the only tea they served. Our beloved iced tea was no more. Not only was the cold drink missing in action, but also the ice. There was no ice served in cafés or restaurants.

We began our jobs in earnest; our son waiting patiently for school to resume after the NZ summer holiday, our daughter landing a job in a laboratory, and my wife began her medical practice. I was cutting my teeth on a project with adolescent mental health; located in a public service unit attached to the large public hospital. I was supporting the development of a family therapy program, but the tracking system was not yet in the picture.

A meeting in Phoenix, Arizona, hosted by the Milton Erickson Foundation to honor Jay Haley, was the beginning of the New Zealand connection. At the reception, I met two family therapists who had moved to New Zealand some years before. We discussed my visiting New Zealand and perhaps doing a workshop. I said, "I could spare two weeks." They put me in touch with Michael Rimm, a child psychiatrist, who was the clinical director of the public clinic for children and adolescents in South Auckland. He said that the cultural and mental health system and the associated problems were so complex, and even daunting, that six months would be the minimum one should commit.

New Zealand is a tiny country of, now, five million people, far away from everything except Australia and various tiny islands. Indeed, one would expect that the problems that befall their young people would be minimized or at least readily controllable. However, New Zealand, at that time, had the largest teenage suicide rate in the developed world (United Press International, 2004) and one of the highest teen pregnancy rates (UNICEF, 2001). Additionally, some medical illnesses were far worse in New Zealand than in the United States: childhood meningitis, rheumatic fever, asthma, and certain skin diseases such as eczema (Mills et al., 2002). Furthermore, these problems and diseases were proportionally higher in the Māori population (Edmonds et al., 2000; Simmons & Voyle, 2003).

My family came for a six-month period as mentioned, fully expecting to return to the United States afterward. While the acculturation was not easy, we were all happy in New Zealand and decided to extend our commitment. Over time, our lives and careers evolved and life in New Zealand became permanent.

As the adolescent project ended, the unit reorganized and they changed direction, moving away from family therapy. I was recruited to join the Māori Mental Health Services, part of the Auckland Public Health System.

Attending Rosh Hashanah services, I found myself talking to a member of the Synagogue after services, a very large Māori man with a dulcet voice. He was interested in my work as a psychiatrist and family therapist and began heavily touting a position to me that was available in his organization: Clinical Director of Māori Mental Health Services. Working fast, by the next day, I had received an invitation from him to come for an interview and meet his team. He explained that in the Māori culture, when interviewing for a job/position, support people, whom I would choose, should accompany me. This is based on two complementary concepts of cultural competence and cultural safety. "Competence" is a set of congruent behaviors, attitudes, and policies that come together in a system or agency and enable professionals to work effectively in cross-culture situations (Cross et al., 1989). "Safety" is the idea that the other person, be it a client or a colleague, feels safe in the context given their cultural background. In New Zealand workplaces and organizations today, "cultural safety programs" must be practiced; the job interview signals the beginning. Bringing a support person or group of people is promoted and expected. I was reminded of this expectation and was also told to prepare my song, a *waiata*; this would honor and show respect for those who have spoken. It was this later request that stunned me. A song for a job interview? Reflecting on the countless times I had interviewed for positions, I had never been asked to sing. I sought counsel from my family, and my dear 15-year-old son, at the time, suggested that if I sang a song my chances of being hired were slim to none. The unfiltered words of this sweet teenager were convincing. I would recite a poem, instead, which was an option. I was considering one of my favorites, "Dover Beach," by Matthew Arnold. Its immortal last line, "Where ignorant armies clash by night," said it all—the Iraq War was raging. Now my wife wanted to add her perspective. "This poem is not a good idea; Māori people spent many years warring with others and they might take affront." I drove to the interview with my supports: a dignified Māori elder statesman and a Māori woman who had left the law and instead worked directly with children, her face tattooed with the traditional Māori moko. A third colleague accompanied the group; she was a clinician, mother to eight children, with a beautiful singing voice. Since I was still feeling wobbly about my own singing, it was comforting to have her there. We four walked into the room, seeing two parallel lines of chairs; one across from the other, with the staff from the organization seated along the one line, with the kaumatua (Māori elder) in the first chair, like an orchestra; and the second line for my entourage. The welcoming ceremony, the pōwhiri, was begun with a karakia, a prayer. As each staff member spoke in te reo Māori, the customary waiata (song) was sung to show respect to the speaker. Once all their staff had spoken, and welcomed us, then it was our turn to introduce ourselves, each one of us speaking, followed by a waiata.

On my drive to this meeting, I recalled a Hebrew prayer called the Shema (Hear, O Israel: the Lord is our God, The Lord is one). This solumn central prayer, is inclusive of all monotheistic religions. It was quite brief and could be chanted easily—carrying a tune was not necessary. Surprisingly, I stood and chanted with ease. When we had all spoken, the parallel seating was changed and a circle was created as each side walked slowly toward the other for the official greeting, the hongi. Men pressing their foreheads and noses together and women being kissed on the cheek—sharing breath cements the pledges that had been made. The final act of breaking bread together, kai, concluded the meeting. Within a few days, I was officially the new Clinical Director.

The attention given to ritual and process by the Māori people is in stark contrast to American culture. With an apparent insouciance for the clock, every meeting and therapy session begins and ends with a karakia, prayer, and sometimes waiata (song). While this might generate considerable angst for the efficiency experts in US clinics, it boldly pronounces that among the Māori, ritual is highly valued. These rituals, whose purpose I slowly grasped, were essential to community building.

My directorship at Māori Mental Health was a valuable experience; I felt honored by my inclusion into their families and community, but the chronicity of this heavily medicated patient group challenged me to make changes. I loved their focus on *whakapapa* (the family lineage); that was music to my ears. I learned that in the Māori culture, your identity is based by your ancestral background and not your vocational role. Referring to a friend as "close bones" is when your ancestors are buried close to each other. Together with Maori senior nurse, Rachel, we set about trying to make changes; she guided me along the way.

These chronically mentally ill patients with files two feet deep were seen by most as hopeless. When I consulted with them, I could not understand why they were not contributing members of society while still under care. Many had hidden skills and work experience; there was real potential. With a job, they could transform their crippling patient identity and ascend to a richer life.

The inactivity of this patient population, along with their medications, caused significant weight gain and led to obesity. Rachel and I began an exercise and nutrition program, led by a personal trainer from a prestigious gym in an affluent part of town. She volunteered her time, feeling an obligation to her Māori community. She was a breath of fresh air, creating an empowering narrative based on the Māori legacy of courage and vitality. The patients attended faithfully.

When we actively began initiating the "jobs program" for our consumers, with the local non-profit group, there was resistance. Our manager said, "Jobs are not our responsibility; our role is to give our patients medications." This was more than a disappointment, it was an obvious permanent stone wall. New to the country and this community, I would never find the supports to move any stones, not least of all a wall. I reluctantly resigned from my position; I could not continue to maintain, in good faith, the hopeless viewpoint. The patients needed more.

I accepted a position at Windsor House, as Clinical Director of a national residential program for severely troubled youth; I felt at home. I had missed working with children and adolescents. This was the opportunity I had longed for since my frustration working in Philadelphia, where services were based on capacity rather than excellence. Here was my chance to design an effective adolescent treatment program.

Within a short period, there it was again; the organization needed cost-effective therapy and, as importantly, an efficient way of tracking outcomes so that clinicians' efforts and outcomes could be measured.

Absent that, we would continue to disappoint our children and their families. We adopted the results-based accountability (RBA) framework to develop a front-line outcome-tracking system. This framework had transformed governmental systems worldwide; it was the innovation that fueled my optimism and our performance. In addition, we streamlined Intensive Structural Therapy (IST), to be more data focused.

1

THE BROKEN PROMISES OF FAMILY THERAPY
THE FATAL FLAW

In the rare moments when 15-year-old Scott opened up, he confided that he has always been lonely. He was removed from his family as an infant by New Zealand social services because of his mother's drug habit; over the years, he would return to Mom only for brief interludes. He had many caregivers in his short life. His biological dad had been in and out of prison for most of Scott's childhood. Scott entered our residential program for severely troubled adolescents after a string of burglaries followed by a car theft and a high-speed car chase that reportedly exceeded 100 mph in a residential neighborhood.

Scott is the youngest of his mother's six children with his father. His parents' fractious relationship is periodically interrupted by his father's incarcerations, as well as by their interludes with other partners with whom they also have children. Initially, Scott's mother was reluctant to engage with our program, and when she discovered that our family therapist had contacted Scott's father, she severed all contact. Scott's 21-year-old brother, however, was willing to work with us.

DOI: 10.4324/9781003161257-2

Meeting Scott, one would be surprised by his affability, given his destructive history. He presented a tidy appearance with a welcoming smile. He was a talented artist and excelled at sports, especially rugby. He had no remorse, however, for his string of burglaries and car chases; he was cavalier regarding any possible vehicular danger to himself or innocent bystanders.

I have met many Scotts during my 16-year tenure with Windsor House. Thirty-two adolescents were residing in the one-year program when I stepped into the position. The vast majority were behaviorally identical to Scott. We had one source of referrals: the social service offices from across New Zealand. The residential setting was a former camp on many acres; previously, it had been a beautiful pastoral landscape. It was in stark contrast to the strife and poverty from which the majority of our children hailed. Our program was a brief respite from these mean streets. These adolescents were all too soon returning to their communities and anguished families. The simple goal should be to help these young people have happy, socially constructive lives.

While we and the other social agencies were the trustworthy backdrops for these children, they idealized a permanent emotional succorance from their families and, frankly, so did we. Our first order of business was family engagement. The IST model was well suited to this approach.

I advanced this model, with its foundational component of structural family therapy (SFT), which was developed in the 1960s. I was purposeful in choosing the word "intensive"; I wanted to knock on the door of complacency and urge therapists to intervene on the interactional patterns that could lead to faster change. A parent who repeatedly bails out his delinquent son, whereby the young person has no consequence to his behavior, is the homeostatic maintainer (HM) of the system and this maintains the status quo; the system is "stuck." IST mandates that clinicians perturb the family system to reveal the HM to bring about fast change.

When I accepted my position at Windsor House, the individual psychodynamic model prevailed; family therapy was absent, nowhere to be found. Their clinical work was based on a Jungian-influenced sand tray treatment, where the therapist encouraged the client to express themselves using sand, water, and miniature objects (Sandplay Therapists of America, n.d.). These youngsters all came from embattled families in impoverished communities; the sand trays along with the one-to-one psychoanalytic therapy were "fiddling while Rome burned." Addressing systemic change would rebuild their houses.

Sixty years ago, family therapy had so much vitality and efficacy that it looked set to take over the clinical world. It did not sit on the periphery. As I mentioned, there were two professors modernizing psychiatry during my residency training: Aaron Beck, founder of CBT, and Salvador Minuchin, founder of SFT. Beck's model, considered innovative, was a variation of individual therapy, the prevailing paradigm of the time. He posited that behavior is modified by changing one arm of a triangle that consists of behavior, cognition, and emotions. According to Beck, changing the cognition causes changes in the other two domains and mitigates the presenting problem. This conceptualization paved the way for this widely used model of individual psychotherapy. CBT was not paradigmatically transformative. It continued to focus on the individual, as had its psychoanalytic predecessors.

By comparison, Dr. Minuchin's model was radically new, a genuine "paradigm shift" in the tradition of T. S. Kuhn, who coined this phrase. The "patient," according to Minuchin, was the family system. He taught us that "mind" (consciousness) is a manifestation of context; the result of an individual's history, cognitive apparatus, and most importantly, the contemporary context that brings forth expressed tenets of the self. Treatment addresses the *extracorporeal mind*, that is, the influential people in a client's social ecology. These relationships were likely maintaining the problem.

Systems theory is the theoretical foundation of family therapy (Minuchin, 1998). Gregory Bateson said that systems are like Russian dolls—"a system within a system within a system... where figures nest" (personal communication, 1979). Like the dolls, family systems are connected and nested.

A system is not just any old collection of things; it is a set of elements that are coherently organized in a way such that it achieves a goal (Meadows, 2008). Families are but one example of such a system.

> In the case of drug addiction, an individual's abuse of drugs is not seen as (only) their issue. Thus it does not matter how loving and supportive a family is toward the drug user because their good intentions will not cure the abuser. Moreover, the drug abuser with a strong desire and motivation cannot resolve their difficulties alone. The individual's addiction can only be treated once everyone recognizes that it is a subset of a more extensive system of influences and societal issues.
>
> (Meadows, 2008).

From our clinical family systems perspective, the family needs to do more than appreciate their involvement; members must change to "cure" the addict by restructuring their family system.

Shortly after Salvador Minuchin passed away in 2017, I published an audio blog in which I suggested that this pioneering therapist was also a brilliant scientist. He had introduced to psychotherapy the concept of "structure," empowering clinicians to assess a family system from the observable interactions of closeness and distance against the backdrop of the developmental stages of the family members. The proximity and distance between a father and son when the boy is three years of age are very different from the closeness between them when the young man is 18. The beauty of this model, when assessing family structure, forecasts the functionality of the family.

Introduction to Psychosomatic Research

Princeton professor, T. S. Kuhn, a physicist and philosopher of science, published in 1962 the book *The Structure of Scientific Revolutions*. This groundbreaking book, considered a landmark in intellectual history, was where he introduced the concept of "paradigm shift," dramatically revising how scientists view the progression of scientific theories. Previously, it was believed that the scientific method was steady, cumulative progress. Kuhn, however, saw a set of normal and revolutionary phases leading to conceptual breakthroughs that would challenge how science should work. There was a belief that scientists gathered data on which they constructed a theory; Kuhn said it was the other way around. The scientist postulated the theory, and then the scientist sought confirmation from observing and experimenting with this explanatory framework. Fifty years ago, Minuchin et al. (1978) sought confirmation of their paradigm that the locus of the problem resided in the immediate context of the family. When the child is triangulated, the child becomes symptomatic, serving a function in the family system; it diffuses the parental conflict. With the introduction of video technology, family therapists observed their videoed sessions and detected this clear pattern. When there was stress between the parents (the parental dyad), the child activated. This research, using physiological markers, confirmed the scientific theory of the family as a dynamic system/unit where the symptom stabilized the family.

Minuchin's confirmation of his paradigm is in the form of grounded, physical findings; this approach stands out in the area of mental health, where so much flimsy theoretical substantiation is subjective responses to queries. This provided a solid foundation to develop a most effective treatment for psychosomatic conditions; moving the field of family therapy into mainstream psychiatry at the time.

Minuchin and Bernice Rosman, his collaborating psychologist, tested the validity of their psychosomatic model and published the findings in the book *Psychosomatic Families* (1978). Their methodology, the Family Interactional Task, generated observable scientific data. In this exercise, the family sat around a table and responded to pre-recorded queries asked by a tape player. The questions were designed to detect family interactional patterns hypothesized to maintain psychosomatic symptomatology. From this perspective, the family's interactions, rather than the individual child, were the "patient" being assessed.

The family responded to queries such as "Discuss a recent family conflict." While psychosomatic families struggled to answer this query, control families showed no problems in responding. Graduate students coded the videos of these sessions, blinded to the families. Their findings showed significantly different interactional patterns in the psychosomatic families. These data were reliable; these grounded interactions were spontaneous, observable responses to one another, not mediated by the researcher. This early research demonstrated that structural family therapy discovered characteristic structures.

The second part of the study, the diagnostic stress interview, was designed to determine if the psychosomatic family interactional patterns led to diabetic ketoacidosis in juvenile diabetic youngsters presenting to the Children's Hospital of Philadelphia. Minuchin's team postulated three discrete categories of these young people who manifested extreme lability. One group consisted of children with out-of-control diabetes because of medical factors. The second group, deemed "behavioral diabetics," were children who deliberately manipulated their diabetic regimen for secondary gain (i.e., gorging themselves with sugar in the evening, becoming symptomatic, and thus being excused from school the next day). The third group was deemed "psychosomatic diabetics." The families of these young people were different; they manifested certain interactional family patterns that exacerbated their children's symptomatology. In this third group, the researchers postulated that these psychosomatic family interactions were pathognomonic for these youngsters' out-of-control diabetes (Minuchin et al., 1978, pp. 22–29) (Figures 1.1–1.4).

In part two of the study design, the child and both parents had intravenous needles through which aliquots of blood were withdrawn at regular intervals. The interview was divided into four periods. During the first two periods, the child was outside the room, observing his parents through a one-way mirror. Following a baseline discussion in which the parents spoke about neutral topics, the parents were then asked in Period I to discuss problems in the family. In Period II, the interviewer entered and exacerbated stress by siding with one parent against the other. During

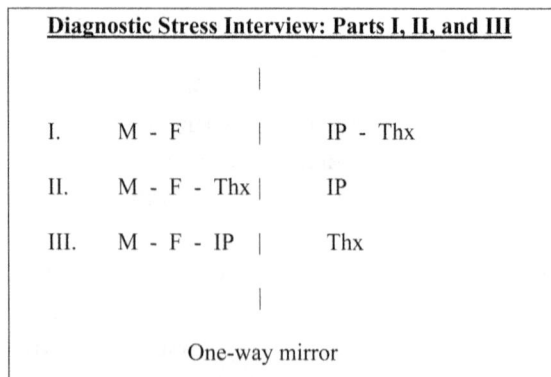

Diagnostic Stress Interview: Parts I, II, and III		
	|	
I.	M - F |	IP - Thx
II.	M - F - Thx |	IP
III.	M - F - IP |	Thx
	|	
	One-way mirror	

Figure 1.1 Diagrammatic presentation of the schedule of the three active periods of the diagnostic stress interview.

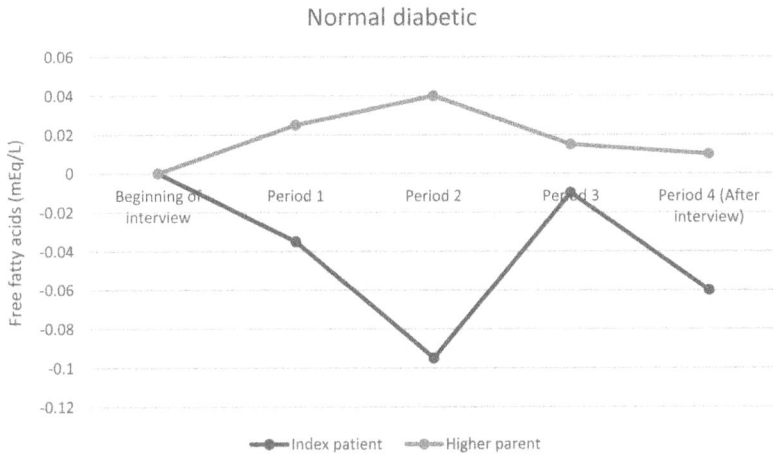

Figure 1.2 Families' free fatty acids (FFA) during the diagnostic stress interview: "Normal diabetic" families.

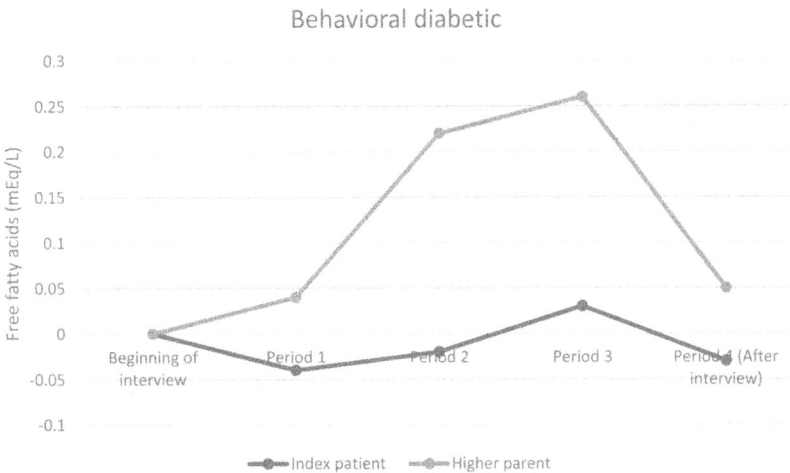

Figure 1.3 Families' free fatty acids during the diagnostic stress interview: "Behavioral diabetic" families.

Period III, the child came into the room and the interviewer left. In this part, a characteristic transactional pattern is observed in psychosomatic families. The parents diffused their conflict by involving their child. As the parents' free fatty acids fell, the child's rose even more steeply. Period IV was a turn-off period, in which the family related alone in a room.

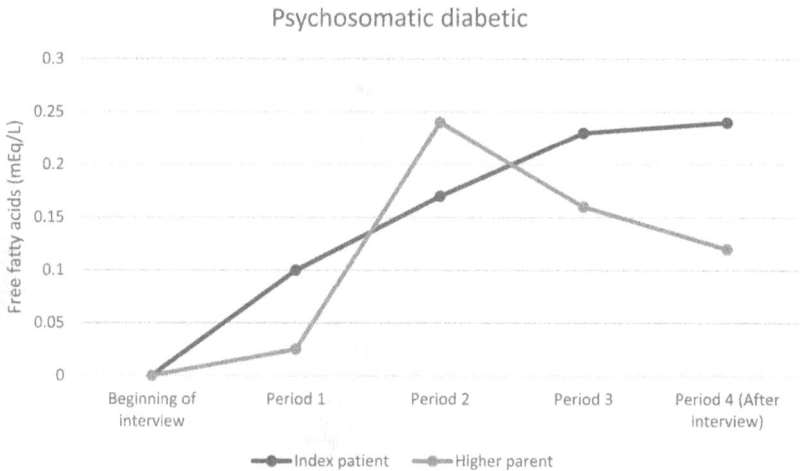

Figure 1.4 Families' free fatty acids during the diagnostic stress interview: "Psychosomatic diabetic" families.

If one assumes that free fatty acids correlate with stress, then the triangulation can be seen as serving a function for the system. In Periods III and IV, the triangulation relieved the stress that the parents were experiencing. However, the cost to the child was demonstrated in terms of the rise of their free fatty acids and the ensuing symptomatology. This indicated the interrelationship between the child's physiology and the family interactions, evidencing family functioning as an integrated unit.

The findings of this study supported Minuchin's postulation of a third group, psychosomatic diabetics with specific interactional patterns. When triangulated, the diabetic child becomes ketotic, requiring hospitalization.

Dr. Lester Baker, the diabetologist involved in this research, related the following anecdote to me. The physicians at the children's hospital called him and said they had a 12-year-old girl who was losing weight and they could find no medical cause. They asked if the PCGC psychosomatic researchers would evaluate her psychologically to see if her symptoms were psychosomatic. The family was assessed with the Family Interactional Task and did not manifest the characteristics of a psychosomatic family: there was no conflict avoidance, overprotectiveness, enmeshment, triangulation, or rigidity. Minuchin's group called the pediatrician and reported the results: the girl was not losing weight on this psychological basis. The team suggested that the hospital would need to do further investigations. The girl was found to have a pineal tumor.

With reflection, I mused, I had come a long way from the verbal sparring in philosophy classes I experienced in college. This was scientific inquiry in front of me with observable data.

Over the decades, these basic principles of the Psychosomatic Model have been pivotal to my clinical work. For example, interactional patterns like triangulation are ubiquitous, not only in psychosomatic families but in most troubled families.

With research and scientific data, I was optimistic in the early days that the family therapy paradigm had a great future ahead of it. As a field, we were poised to make significant progress to become the mental health treatment of choice.

We are now many years from the time when the courageous founders first ventured to work with families. Family therapy certainly has made vital and significant progress, with large organizations such as the American Association of Marriage and Family Therapy (AAMFT) with 25,000 members and professional degrees such as master's (MFT) and PhDs in family therapy. The well-known Maudsley method of family-based treatment (FBT) for working with juvenile anorexia nervosa is based on Minuchin's model, as are multisystemic therapy (MST) and functional family therapy (FFT). Using these formalized protocols, clinicians apply "systems thinking" to engage successfully with troubled families in their communities. Family therapists across the world from the US, the Americas, Europe and Asia, committed, skilled clinicians provide invaluable service. But I am still concerned for our field. Despite the advancements, family therapy is increasingly marginalized. In a survey of over 2,000 psychotherapists in the United States and Canada, Cook et al. (2010) observed that only 17% of clinicians in the total sample considered themselves first and foremost as "family therapists." Moreover, concerning the clientele, 84% of clinicians reported that they primarily work with individuals, while only 9% reported families as their primary type of client. Interestingly, 49% of clinicians reported that they made use of a "family systems" approach in therapy, which was second only to cognitive-behavioral therapy (around 80%). These findings may imply that psychotherapists are happy to conceptualize difficulties in terms of the family but are less enthusiastic about actually working with families. That is not family therapy. Even more worrying is the notion that in a US national survey of psychotherapists calling themselves "marriage and family therapists," CBT remained the most frequently endorsed therapeutic approach (Northey, 2002).

Even more worrisome, Heatherington et.al,2012 surveyed, 80% of Ph.D. programs designated as "clinical science" programs endorsed a cognitive-behavioral orientation, compared to 17% endorsement of "family systems" as a theoretical orientation. Of all other Ph.D. programs surveyed at "comprehensive universities," 67% identified a cognitive-behavioral orientation compared to a 20% endorsement of family systems. In Psy.D. programs surveyed from universities, 48% endorsed CBT as a theoretical orientation and 16% family systems; further, Psy.D. programs and Ph.D. programs from "freestanding professional schools," 32% endorsed CBT and 22% identified family systems as a theoretical orientation.

CBT was one of the main competitors of family therapy. Using a blunt measure of database searches from 2010–2019, there were 10.8 million articles relating to CBT and 3.64 million relating to family therapy. While not reflecting the quality of the researched contributions, this does, however, serve as a measure of the vitality of a movement concerning scholarly work. Sadly, family therapy has fallen far behind. Evidence-based literature is the currency of decision makers in large government systems, many academic programs, and managed care companies. The widespread understanding that CBT has the most extensive evidence base often makes it the first choice treatment in the field of psychotherapy. Does it deserve its jeweled crown?

Although the American Psychological Association task force lists CBT as the only treatment with strong research support for almost 80% of psychological disorders, Leichsenring and Steinert (2017) argue that, under scrutiny, flaws are visible in its research base. A recent meta-analysis found that only 17% of 144 randomized, controlled trials (RCTs) of CBT were "of appropriate scientific rigor" (Leichsenring & Steinert, 2017). Another meta-analysis revealed that CBT achieved a large effect size only in comparison with waiting list conditions. The authors concluded that the additional gains of CBT may indeed be limited to the allegiance effects with therapists (Leichsenring & Steinert, 2017).

Although a first-line treatment should be clearly more effective than any other treatment, Leichsenring and Steinert (2017) suggest that due to the inconsistency among CBT research, there is no "clear" evidence that CBT is superior to any of its psychotherapeutic competitors in treating depression and anxiety-based disorders. That CBT is the psychotherapy standard of care is called in question. With Scott's chaotic situation, his conduct disorder, and complex family, it seems incomprehensible that an individual's cognition could have sufficient jurisdiction to transform this chaos.

In reviewing family medicine journals and periodicals, I found that when a psychotherapy was mentioned, it was almost invariably CBT. It was reported to me by a colleague who attended a Harvard conference on psychopharmacology that, at one point, the chair of the meeting stated, "For those interested in psychotherapy, we have a CBT clinician available for consultation," suggesting that psychotherapy equates to CBT. In the periodical *Evidence-Based Practice*, a highly regarded journal for family medical practitioners, many articles that introduce psychological treatments often limit their consideration to CBT. I asked myself, "Where is family therapy in family medicine?" The hegemony of CBT's status tends to limit the reception of other models in the workforce.

Evidence-based medicine (EBM), defined as medical practice informed by research, has not, for the most part, helped the family therapy movement. It is widely considered to have saved millions of lives, but it serves as a gatekeeper to new ideas and innovation. Government agencies and HMOs look for the security and protection of EBM programs to shield them from criticism and litigation. This is unfortunate. I've seen effective, community-based family treatment programs passed over because they missed the imprimatur of EBM.

Psychotropic medications have also contributed to family therapy's marginalization. It is easy for doctors to prescribe medicines as a simple answer, asking no further questions, to avoid the messiness of their patients' lives. Antidepressant use in the United States has risen dramatically over the past few decades (Kantor et al., 2015), and even ten years ago, the country was spending at least two billion dollars a year prescribing antidepressants (Chen et al., 2008). Prescriptions for antidepressants increased a staggering 10% per annum in the United Kingdom between 1998 and 2012 (Ilyas & Moncrief, 2012). The question in pharmacotherapy is: What can we alter in your brain chemistry? In systems work, the crucial question is: Who or what is depressing you?

According to Dr. Craig Whittington and colleagues of the National Collaborating Centre for Mental Health, London, antidepressants are no more effective than a placebo for mild to moderate depression (Whittington et al., 2004). The British National Health Service's guidelines recommend that antidepressants should not be used as a first line for mild to moderate depression; yet, as we all know, they are more widely used (Whittington et al., 2004).

Community/family doctors should be advocating for an available family therapist—someone who can transform the contextually generated dysphoria of their patients, rather than the false hope of medications. The billions spent in the public mental health systems to address the severely troubled youngsters mentioned in these chapters often go toward treatment with medications resulting in no systemic change. Like CBT, medications will not address the context of these youngsters, especially when adding the complications of systemic racism and poverty. These social problems are daunting and often lead to significant family stress. It is the war at the heart of the family that elevates young people above clinical thresholds.

The splintered field of family therapy has considerable responsibility in contributing to its marginalization. Since its inception, the field has divided into many diverse schools. In a comprehensive article, Evan Imber-Black (2014) explains the origins and early "model wars" of the family therapy field. She elucidates the relevant factors in the development of the field over the past decades; in short, her message indicates that we rode off in all directions. What remains unclear is why family therapists were so motivated to "jump ship" and embrace new models, such as the Cybernetic and Milan models in the late 1970s and 1980s, and then more contemporaneously, narrative therapy. I find scant evidence that the migration of models was based on improved clinical outcomes.

Over the years, I have mused that family therapy is like Madison Avenue fashion, with its randomly changing hemlines. Mysteriously, family therapy theories seem to come to prominence based on factors other than their effectiveness. Trendiness is not what our clients need; they deserve a scientific commitment to good results.

Narrative therapy is a widely practiced model. Among its leading theorists are David Epston and the late Michael White. The therapy purports to help people identify their values, skills, and knowledge, so they can confront their problems. The therapist helps the client to co-author a new personal narrative by investigating their history. Narrative therapy claims to be a social justice approach to therapeutic conversations, seeking to challenge dominant discourses that shape people's lives in destructive ways (Morgan, 2000). Putting aside my many questions about this individual approach, more importantly, it does not appear to ameliorate the presenting problems according to Busch, who found minimal evidence of its effectiveness (Busch, 2011). There is an immediacy and urgency to a family's escalating problems, and narrative therapy's high value of social justice does not translate that value into what ails the struggling family.

The mindfulness movement is increasingly prevalent. PBS NewsHour reported on a program that was teaching mindfulness techniques to children in the inner city (PBS NewsHour, 2014). The personal benefits of mindfulness for children are apparent (Bögels et al., 2008; Singh et al., 2007); however, these inner-city youngsters are, in many cases, likely to be going home to intense poverty and no dinner. This is a big ask for these young children, even if they find a safe place in their minds, to gird themselves from the bedlam of their families' lives.

The failure of the family therapy leaders to unite was their persistent focus on process and its compelling allure; it paralyzed the field. The "model wars," as described by Imber-Black (2014), blinded the creators and they disregarded the imperative of committing to models that provided the best outcomes.

This practice may well have been a disadvantage in building an evidence-base; the field it did not appear to learn and mimic what allowed cognitive-behavioral rivals to be so effective. Had the field of family ther-apy, rallied together around simple, fundamental theories of change and attempted to market (as Beck and his contemporaries did) user friendly interventions, the current evidence-based climate might be considerably more balanced.

2

CHALLENGING EVIDENCE-BASED MEDICINE

THE AGE OF SKEPTICISM: STUDIES THAT DEFINE THE STANDARD OF CARE ARE UNRELIABLE

Evidence-based medicine (EBM), a term attributed to David Sackett (Claridge & Fabian, 2005), is an approach to medical practice intended to optimize decision-making by emphasizing the use of "current best evidence" (Sackett, 1997) from well-designed and well-constructed research. The general idea of making use of scientific knowledge in patient care first caught the attention of researchers and clinicians in 1972 following the publication of the classic text, *Effectiveness and Efficiency: Random Reflections on Health Services* (Cochrane, 1972). Archie Cochrane's report led to randomized controlled trials (RCTs), the basis of the EBM movement, where treatments are applied variously to randomly selected patients in order to compare their effects being held up as the best research model.

In the transitional period, from 1900 to the 1970s, textbooks and peer-reviewed journals were the convenient vehicles for scientific knowledge. In the modern era of EBM, computerized databases and the internet have allowed access to the results of RCTs, the main tool of choice (Claridge & Fabian, 2005).

DOI: 10.4324/9781003161257-3

The basic tenets of EBM are quite comforting: always try to apply scientific evidence to practice, always try to assess the quality of evidence (i.e., relevant risks and benefits of treatment or lack thereof), always be conscientious, and explicitly and judiciously use the current "best evidence" when making decisions about individual patient care.

Many aspects of medical care, however, depend on individual factors, such as quality and value-of-life judgments, that often do not yield to scientific methods. EBM, on the other hand, seeks to clarify those parts of medical practice that can be objectified. These are then subjected to scientific methodology in an attempt to best predict possible medical treatment outcomes.

EBM consists of three distinct, but interdependent areas: treatment, systematic reviews, and meta-reviews. In treating patients, medical practitioners should select treatment options based on the "best available research" for their patients with acute or chronic pathologies. These studies should be human-centered and be published in refereed journals. Systematic reviews provide a broader overview of available knowledge on specific topics. The introduction of EBM was transformative and claimed the status of a "medical movement" that works to popularize the methodology and usefulness of data to the public, communities, educational institutions, and continuing education of practicing professionals. A new culture was created such that procedures and interventions now required more rigorous supportive evidence.

EBM Critiques

Over the years, there have been several general critiques and concerns about EBM. It has become more difficult to compare the patient in studies with the patient in the consultation room. The applications of EBM to populations where data is pooled and aggregated challenge the individual clinician. The large RCTs are useful for examining discrete interventions for carefully defined medical conditions, but with more complexity seen in patients (severity of condition, comorbid conditions), the more difficult it is to assess these treatment effects. EBM guidelines do not extrapolate problems that occur with different populations or longer timeframes. More specifically, even if several top-quality studies are available, questions remain as to how far and to which populations the results are "generalizable" to (Gomory, 2013). There are some unresearched areas due to ethical considerations such as open-heart surgical procedures. Some groups have been historically under-researched (racial minorities and people with comorbid diseases); therefore, the literature is sparse in areas that do not allow for generalizing. Trials that may be considered "gold standard" (i.e., randomized, double-blind, placebo-controlled trials) are expensive, so funding sources play a role in what is investigated. Public authorities may fund preventive medicine studies to improve public health, in general, while pharmaceutical companies may support studies intended to demonstrate the efficacy and safety of their particular drugs. According to Gomory, EBM itself has never been evaluated in a controlled Cochrane Library protocol. In other words, EBM has not been validated: Gomory asks (Gomory, 2013), do practitioners who use EBM get better outcomes than those who do not use it? Moreover, as mentioned, while EBM may be able to predict the "best treatment" for an average population, it may be less practical for individuals who are in an unpredictable environment outside of the test environment (Gomory, 2013). There is the risk that RCTs are too imprecise to be effective in overly complicated mental health treatment programs. Therefore, despite the focus on quantitative data, meta-analysis tends to be less discriminatory, accepting the data at face value rather than questioning how it was collected (Goodman, 1999). Quantitative data lacks specificity, which means it can be quite tricky to combine EBM with clinical judgment and patient wishes. The mere definition of an EBM "expert" is often subjectively defined, making it hard to determine who is and who isn't an expert on this methodology (Goodman, 1999).

It is important to note that evidence-based practices tend to be defined through consensus. In other words, these tenets may focus on the political implications—not the scientific progress. It is true that EBM has a prominent place but the influence of qualitative approaches (i.e., case studies) may be absent. These should be encouraged, primarily because many of the past century's most notable medical discoveries have occurred as a result of observations—not experimentation (Goodman, 1999).

Other more contemporary problems with EBM are the tarnishing of EBM's "brand" due to vested interests (i.e., pharmaceutical industries have a history of defining what constitutes an illness, what counts as a risk state, and who funds and manages empirical studies, while the government has been known to distort research data for political purposes). Now here we are with large data sets, unmanageable amounts of data, and an abundance of clinical guidelines that need to be refreshed/ rewritten daily. The statistically significant results can appear to "overestimate" real-life benefits, whose harmful side-effects can overshadow any real benefits. This overestimation and overshadowing can, and often does, lead to noticeable shifts in treatment, from disease care to risk management. As a result of this overestimation, there is a shift toward algorithmic rules rather than individual care, which may have the risk of turning health care into a mechanical, uncaring process. Many argue that there is an incompatibility; EBM is a poor fit for patients with complicated real-life situations that feature multiple issues (Greenhalgh et al., 2014).

Enter John Ioannidis: Physician, Statistician, Skeptic

There are increasing challenges to the published medical research, even in the most prestigious journals. Stanford professor John Ioannidis offers some of the most compelling arguments. Dr. Ioannidis applied rigorous statistical analysis to what seemed to him a "sloppy field" (Freedman 2010b). David H. Freedman, writing in *The Atlantic*, quotes Ioannidis as saying, "I assumed that everything we physicians did was right, and I was going to help verify it. All we'd have to do was systematically review the evidence, trust what it told us, and then everything would be perfect" (Freedman, 2010b). Soon into this quest, Ioannidis began questioning the statistics in some of these esteemed journals, such as *Nature* and *The New England Journal of Medicine*. He found that *as much as 90% of the published medical information that doctors rely on is flawed: either misleading, exaggerated, or sometimes simply wrong due to research error (Freedman, 2010b).*

Ioannidis was struck by how many findings of all types were refuted by later studies. Indeed, he found that though RCTs were less likely to be retracted, nevertheless, one-fourth of RCTs were still later refuted, and successful attempts at study replication are uncommon. He attributed this phenomenon primarily to a lack of statistical power, and prevailing bias in study design (Ioannidis, 2005). Throughout the 2000s, Ioannidis and his team conducted quantitative statistical meta-analyses of literature across medical science (Ioannidis et al., 2001; Ioannidis, 2003) and ultimately concluded that the entirety of EBM was subject to flaws of serious concern (Ioannidis, 2005). For example, in multi-center studies, researchers found that mammograms, colonoscopies, and prostate-specific antigen (PSA) tests were far less useful than had been claimed. And the widely prescribed antidepressants, such as Prozac, Zoloft, and Paxil, were shown to be less effective than placebos, in spite of considerable earlier research that had supported their effectiveness (Freedman, 2010b).

Ioannidis found the range of errors being committed daunting: what questions the researchers asked, how they set up the studies, which patients they recruited, and how they analyzed the data, along with how they presented the results and how particular subjects came to be published in medical journals were among the many errors. He found that "80 percent of non-randomized studies (by far the most common type) turn out to be wrong, as do 25 percent of supposedly gold-standard randomized trials, and as much as 10 percent of the platinum-standard large randomized trials" (Freedman, 2010b). A third to a half of the most acclaimed research in medicine was proven untrustworthy.

Ioannidis came to conclude that many "proven" scientific theories are subsequently shown to be either false or exaggerated. This finding belies the idea that evidence-based medical research is the road to scientific truth; Ioannidis found that academic research was more likely to be mistaken than right. In a separate article on Ioannidis, in The New York Times, David Freedman joked, Meteorologists are the only people who get paid to be wrong should be extended to cover all experts (Freedman, 2010a).

Today, Dr. Ioannidis, a professor of Medicine and Health Research and Policy in the Stanford School of Medicine, according to his Stanford bio, has published over 1,000 peer-reviewed articles. His classic article, "Why Most Published Research Findings Are False" (Ioannidis, 2005), has been one of the most accessed articles in the Public Library of Science, with around three million "hits." He continues to hold EBM to account, as in his recent article, "Spin, Bias, and Clinical Utility in Systematic Reviews of Diagnostic Studies" (Ioannidis, 2020).

P-Values: The Decider

When analyzing EBM issues using the "p-value" as a level of statistical significance, it is essential to be cognizant that the p-value is often misunderstood. Generally, a p-value is the likelihood that, if there was no real relationship between two variables, an observed statistical finding would have occurred through chance alone. A p-value of 0.05, therefore, implies that there is only a 5% chance that the observed result would have occurred by chance. The threshold of 5% is used as an arbitrary cut-off point in the majority of studies. Findings are not deemed statistically significant unless there is a less than 5% chance they could have occurred by chance alone. People tend to mistakenly view a significant p-value as proof that a given hypothesis (e.g., this particular drug significantly lowers cholesterol) is true. More importantly, they tend to view a significant p-value as proof that any other possible hypothesis is not true (Goodman, 1999). A statistically significant finding neither proves the truth of a certain hypothesis nor disproves any other explanations for the observed findings. This is why replication of studies is so important within quantitative academia.

Another issue with the p-value is that it does not take into account the magnitude of the effect; therefore a result could be statistically significant but represent only a minor "real-world" effect. In the hypothetical case of a study measuring the efficacy of a new antidepressant drug, there may be a statistically significant result overall, that is, there was an average decrease in people's scores on a depression scale of three points. For clinicians working with their patients/clients, a change of three points on a depression scale is impossible to observe or discern. Likewise, for clients, they may shift three points on a scale without noticing any difference in the way they think or feel. The shift is never fixed. The result, therefore, has little use in the real world.

This use of the 0.05 significance as an arbitrary cut-off incentivizes the manipulation or control of the number of incorrect conclusions produced in a particular investigation. If an initial analysis is insignificant, researchers will revise and re-run experiments going in search of the significant result, rather than accessing the actual implications of their work (Goodman, 1999). A common environment where this process (also known colloquially in academia as "p-hacking") occurs is in pharmaceutical drug trials. Pharmaceutical companies run a plethora of studies and only publish or replicate the design of ones in which the 0.05 threshold is reached. The statistical definition of the p-value ensures that if data are analyzed repeatedly, the likelihood of a false positive result increases dramatically (Cui et al., 1999; Schulz & Grimes, 2005). Furthermore, the "p-value fallacy" espouses that results, even if they are significant in the short term, may not be significant in the long term.

Ironically, this research methodology ("p-values") has dominated the field, despite its apparent flaws. In fact, it continues to be used. In other words, government officials and academic researchers have found it useful to have a quantitative methodology that generates conclusions independent of the researchers, producing findings that appear to be objective (Goodman, 1999). Lastly, this research methodology has caused other research methodologies to be neglected, negatively impacting critical thinking (Goodman, 1999).

Industry Influences

EBM's most fundamental flaw is that industry-funded studies are considered "evidence," despite being severely flawed. The evidence base, as a whole, becomes dually flawed as, typically, only studies that observe the desired result are published (Every-Palmer & Howick, 2014). This results in potentially massive disconnects between what will work best in promoting wellbeing, and what is actually done as treatment. An example is the evidence-based first-line treatment for mental health difficulties in psychopharmacology, which is considered far more effective than psychotherapy. As a result, many clinicians have ceased treating anyone with psychotherapy. This is despite the fact that psychopharmacology is ultimately more expensive and no more effective when evidence is further scrutinized (Every-Palmer & Howick, 2014).

The industry is also more likely to favor sponsor-funded medications over non-sponsored medications. A review, published in The American Journal of Psychiatry, examined 30 studies of industry-sponsored treatments and found that approximately 90% of those studies touted sponsor-funded drugs as the more effective treatments (Heres et al., 2006). An analysis of 397 clinical studies published in a variety of psychiatric journals between 2001 and 2003 revealed that 60% of the named researchers (in the clinical trials) received monetary compensation from pharmaceutical companies or other interested parties, and 47% of the researchers had at least one conflict of interest (Perlis et al., 2005). Researchers who had even one conflict of interest were 4.9 times more likely to report positive results than those who were academically neutral (Perlis et al., 2005).

Pharmaceutical companies also habitually "fake" advisory boards and "independent studies" to bolster the authenticity of their product (Every-Palmer & Howick, 2014). Capitalist ideals hold sway, rather than health interests. The danger of such bias in the evidence base is in some ways "immortal" (Every-Palmer & Howick, 2014) in that, even when new studies or meta-analyses are done to discredit old findings, old studies continue to circulate in the online sphere, proliferating misinformation (Every-Palmer & Howick, 2014).

Pharmaceutical companies then make use of this flawed evidence to directly influence the clinical behavior of doctors. They track and target specific medical practitioners, tailoring their interactions with them, to increase their influence (Fugh-Berman & Ahari, 2007), using the studies their company has funded to legitimize any claims. Subsequently, doctors become the voice of this flawed EBM in the sense that they sing the praises of drug treatments to their patients. Over half rely on the dubious information presented to them by drug representatives when forming opinions of new drugs (Millenson, 2003). The way to counteract these efforts is for doctors to seek information from "unconflicted" sources (Fugh-Berman & Ahari, 2007) but, as Millenson (2003) points out, the majority do not.

There is, of course, EBM that is free of corporate interest. A large source of such evidence is the Cochrane Library, a collection of international, systematic reviews of primary research literature in human health care and health policy. These reviews are internationally recognized as the highest standard in evidence-based health care, investigating the effects of interventions for prevention, treatment, and rehabilitation. One paper compared the results of 24 Cochrane reviews, eight pharmaceutical industry-supported meta-analyses, and seven independent meta-analyses of clinical studies that made drug recommendations. The review found that the Cochrane reviews were of better quality, and more likely to address the potential for biases, than industry-supported publications (Jørgensen et al., 2006). More specifically, industry-supported meta-analyses and supposedly independent meta-analyses made recommendations for drugs without any reservations (i.e., after less thorough examinations), while the Cochrane reviews only made recommendations for drugs after cautious and careful review and analysis (Jørgensen et al., 2006).

The same article notes instances in industry-supported studies where medication dosages were used to manipulate outcomes (i.e., comparing insufficient doses of Clozapine with high doses of Olanzapine). Researchers have also been found to use other "tricks" to manipulate research study outcomes, such as excluding non-responders from maintenance meetings/follow-ups and providing detailed analyses of desired results while ignoring or minimizing undesired ones (Heres et al., 2006).

Peer Review and Statisticians

Did you know that listening to the wildly popular song "When I'm Sixty-Four," by The Beatles, can make you younger? In fact, the journal *Psychological Science* revealed this marvel (Simmons et al., 2011). The authors designed a study in which participants were assigned to listen to The Beatles' classic, or another musical piece, then, as part of an entirely unrelated task, asked to give their birth date. Results indicated that participants were, on average, 18 months younger after listening to "When I'm Sixty-Four" than the alternate track. This has significance, of course, with a p-value at the 0.05 level. Upon inspection, naturally, the study is one that conflates correlation with causation. There was an observed association between age and the music track listened to, but in this situation, it is obvious there can be no causal link (Simmons et al., 2011). In others, it is not so easy to discern. Within that period, when the transmission of results of statistical investigations is translated into real-world understanding, there is room for researchers to select methods that provide them the results they desire or infer more from their results than is pragmatic.

Popular Literature

In the popular literature, there are numerous challenges to medical research. Gratzer (2013) discussed the pervasive unreliability of academic research. He reports on the efforts of drug company Amgen to replicate the results of 53 studies that were considered landmarks in cancer research, even going as far as to cooperate with the original researchers. Despite investing extensively in the project, Amgen was only able to replicate six studies successfully. Another group at Bayer was able to repeat only a quarter of 67 pharmaceutical papers. It is reported that between 2000 and 2010, roughly 80,000 patients took part in clinical trials based on studies that were later retracted because of mistakes in the data (Gratzer, 2013).

In another example, a study documented that while only 2% of researchers admitted to fabricating, falsifying, or modifying data or results at least once, a third confessed to other questionable practices such as dropping data points or altering the methodology in response to pressures from funders, and up to 72% stated that they had observed their colleagues engaging in questionable methods (Fanelli, 2009). An article in The Atlantic (Lam, 2015) suggests a few of the many reasons why these issues arise, including the competitiveness of science and the speculation that when more researchers compete for fewer academic posts, they tend to focus on looking for new exciting findings rather than replicating old studies. This competitiveness also leads to harmful practices such as cherry-picking results to create distorted data. On the journals' side of the process, there is a tendency to only look for "interesting" results, which leads to a disproportionate amount of positive findings being published. According to the same article, the peer-review process is also flawed, as research has shown that reviewers have failed to pick up on intentional mistakes inserted into an article.

Reliability of Data in Psychology

EBM took off in the field for two main reasons: it was supported by senior clinicians who were happy to be challenged, and it empowered younger doctors to question received wisdom (Godlee, 2014). However,

EBM has come under criticism for fueling over-diagnosis and over-treatment. According to *The New York Times*, many psychology findings are not as viable as claimed (Carey, 2015). A now-infamous attempt to reproduce 100 studies in three leading psychology journals found that 60 of the studies did not hold up to retesting (Open Science Collaboration, 2015). Needless to say, this research has troubling implications for current psychological theory.

In psychiatry, there are many questions involving the influence of big pharmaceutical companies in producing questionable data. According to Every-Palmer and Howick (2014), evidence-based medicine is failing due to biased trials and selective publication. They argue that:

> Evidence-based medicine (EBM) was announced in the early 1990s as a "new paradigm" for improving patient care. Yet there is currently little evidence that EBM has achieved its aim. Since its introduction, health care costs have increased while there remains a lack of high-quality evidence suggesting EBM has resulted in substantial population-level health gains.
>
> (Every-Palmer & Howick, 2014)

Manipulation of Results

The manipulation of academic literature by way of publication bias is another major issue for EBM in mental health. The authors also discuss the fact that multiple drug companies were fined for the manipulation of results. In a meta-analysis of antidepressant drug trials, Turner et al. (2008) observed that among 74 Food and Drug Administration (FDA)-registered studies, 31%, accounting for 3,449 study participants, were not published due to the acquisition of commercially undesirable results. Whether and how the studies were published was associated with the study outcome. A total of 37 studies viewed by the FDA as having positive results were published. Studies viewed by the FDA as having negative or questionable results were generally either not published or published in a way that conveyed a positive outcome (Turner et al., 2008).

The current "publish or perish" culture in academia is accused of putting undue pressures on researchers that lead them to partake in dubious

research practices. However, misreported data is not a new phenomenon. A historic study observed similar trends that research trials were
three times more likely to have positive results (Dickersin et al., 1987).
More recent investigations suggest that although the problem is not a
new one, it may be getting worse. The proportion of published positive
results to negative results reportedly increased 22% between 1997 and
2007 (Ioannidis & Trikalinos, 2007).

Retractions

It is estimated that between 2001 and 2010, the annual rate of retractions by academic scientific journals increased by over ten times (He,
2013). This may be because errors and other misdeeds are becoming
more common, because research is now being scrutinized more carefully, or even because of pressure on authors at the mercy of an increased
"publish or perish" culture (He, 2013). A review of 2,047 retractions
found that 21.3% of the withdrawals were due to fundamental error,
while 67.4% stemmed from misconduct including fraud (43.4%) and pla-
giarism (9.8%) (Fang et al., 2012).

Importantly, however, even if these biased outcomes are identified,
the electronic legacy of EBM research leads to the fact that even biased
results tend to linger on past their retractions, either through being cited
in other articles or through electronic copies online (Godlee, 2014).

While this paints a bleak picture of the field, the authors also note
that researchers are being scrutinized more carefully, a process that is
helped by new data-analysis tools and plagiarism-detecting software.
This heightened scrutiny may have a deterrent effect on future research
as the likelihood of misconduct being discovered is increased.

What To Do with All This Flawed Scientific Literature?

One mainstream suggestion in response to these issues regarding
EBM is an argument for a "return to real evidence-based medicine"
(Greenhalgh et al., 2014) involving: a focus on providing top-notch,
ethical care to patients; attaining individualized data that both patients
and clinicians can fully understand; use of expert judgment when

adopting and adhering to a clinical rule; sharing informed decision-making efforts with patients through meaningful conversations; development of a robust clinician-patient relationship, while focusing on the human aspects of care; and highlighting the real benefits of EBM principles at a community level, as evidence that better public health is needed.

The reader might conjecture that over the years, these deficits have surely been remediated. A blog post in 2017 by Dr. Ben Goldacre, a practicing physician, professor, and science journalist, stated that he is a strong advocate of EBM and also one of its severest critics. On his blog, "Bad Science," he posted the text of the written evidence he submitted in March 2017 to the British House of Commons Science and Technology Committee of Inquiry on Research Integrity (Goldacre, 2017). His submission refers to watch guard efforts, like the 2004 statement by the International Committee of Medical Journal Editors, asserting that a clinical trial result will not be published if it is not recorded publicly at the outset (Claridge & Fabian, 2005). This new "rule" may be helpful, although, to date, no real actions have been taken, and breaches are common (Goldacre, 2017). This is a significant problem in the scientific literature. It is so significant that there have been requests to replace peer reviewers with paid experts—accredited specialists in the statistical analysis of research literature (Harris, 2016). In other words, these researchers are advocating that EBM be radically revised.

An editorial in the prestigious *Lancet* medical journal (Horton, 2015) described a medical conference where government-employed health care professionals were not allowed to remark about the large amount of incorrect published literature. Participants who worked for government agencies pleaded for their comments to remain unquoted since the forthcoming UK election meant they were living in "purdah" (Horton, 2015), a state of severe restrictions on the freedom of speech. Why the desperate desire for secrecy? This symposium, on the reproducibility and reliability of biomedical research, touched on one of the most sensitive issues in the sciences today: the idea that something may be fundamentally wrong with one of our greatest human creations. The case against EBM is straightforward: much of the scientific literature may simply be untrue.

Conclusion

We accept the fallibility of the evidence domain. The hoodwinking is not that the emperor has no clothes—he's not even on a horse and yet people are applauding his canter.

I support George Stricker's belief (2006) that we must build a bridge between science and practice. He suggests that this worldwide gap could be closed if clinicians share experiences and insights and their local observations and solutions. Clinicians as researchers promise an alternative to traditional research; the field could expand its jurisdiction of the definition of what is acceptable data. As embedded researchers, we can track and report our front-line outcomes, contributing the "real," evidence (Stricker, 2006).

3

A CASE FOR RESULTS-BASED ACCOUNTABILITY

Scott, the 15-year-old that I discussed earlier, with his sad, struggling, broken down family, nagged at my sense of moral responsibility. There are so many Scotts in my clinical world and likely yours. They deserve happy productive lives with reasonably well-functioning family systems. The money spent on mental health treatment has not penetrated the front line of care and addressed the social determinants for those children like Scott.

The elaborate and expensive mental health infrastructures have become fortresses of unquestioning clinical inertia and have led to troubling statistics. Ringel and Sturm's (2001) adjusted calculations for inflation now estimate that the total cost to the US economy of all childhood emotional and behavioral issues could be as high as US$247 billion per annum (Perou et al., 2013). The Lancet Commission on Global Mental Health and Sustainable Development expects a loss of US$16 trillion to the global economy due to mental disorders in the period 2010–2030 (Patel et al., 2018, cited in Leichsenring et al., 2019).

DOI: 10.4324/9781003161257-4

The microsystems of care find that children who are in residential programs like Windsor House, our program in Auckland, are predominantly growing up in low-income households. These children demonstrate the greatest need for clinical services while they have the highest rates of underutilization of services (Bringewatt & Gershoff, 2010). Financial barriers and limited service access prevent low-income families from receiving mental health treatment from a system in the United States that is already "fragmented, and complex" (Bringewatt & Gershoff, 2010). It appears that the high demand for services among economically disenfranchised communities exacerbates the ineffectiveness of the already overstretched, inefficient systems.

This deficit of services may well lead to the findings that up to 20% of disadvantaged youth develop conduct disorders; about one-third of children with early behavioral problems go on to develop these disorders in adolescence, yet only around 20% of students with severe emotional disturbances receive some clinical intervention (Burns et al., 1995; Coid, 2003; Strein et al., 2003).

Poverty exacerbates the problems. Higher rates of disruptive behavior occur in socially underprivileged areas with higher frequencies of single-parent families. They tend to be families with inconsistent/unstable presence of a parental figure, and families in which a primary caregiver(s) exhibits "substance misuse, psychopathology, marital problems, and poor parenting skills" (Attride-Stirling et al., 2001; Hutchings et al., 2007, p. 678).

Despite these societal barriers, some effective therapeutic models mitigate these problems to some degree. For example, family-based prevention and intervention programs, such as functional family therapy (FFT; Cottrell & Boston, 2002) and multisystemic therapy (MST; Littell et al., 2005) have promising research bases with regard to treating children and adolescents. These programs serve to transform the severe behavioral problems manifested by conduct-disordered young people. Generally, family-based treatments are efficacious in treating a wide range of disorders among young people (Carr, 2014).

This good news goes only so far. The implications of controlled studies do not universally translate into underserved communities. Selecting appropriate intervention strategies becomes increasingly challenging for children and families in low-income-based community mental health clinics due to high incidences of complex and comorbid childhood problems (Harrison et al., 2004; Xue et al., 2005). As such, it is essential to highlight the distinction between efficacious research findings and those that translate into treatment effectiveness in the community.

According to Weisz and Kazdin in 2010, the majority of child psychotherapy literature relies on efficacy studies, which "aims to determine whether a treatment can work," and are "typically conducted under optimal circumstances" (Henggeler & Sheidow, 2012, p. 31). Here, clinicians are highly trained and well supervised, organizational barriers are minimized (such as through the use of university resources), and the selection of clients is limited to those with simple presentations (Schoenwald & Hoagwood, 2001). In contrast, effectiveness studies aim to evaluate the use of a treatment in a realistic setting. In these studies, treatment is conducted by community practitioners in community settings, where clients' complexity can vary, and socioeconomic factors profoundly influence outcomes (Henggeler & Sheidow, 2012). Treatments developed out of efficacy studies seldom work as consistently as intended with complex young people in complicated environments.

Of even more significant concern, numerous researchers question the effectiveness of psychotherapy and pharmacotherapy, which are the key available treatments presently offered to millions of people with mental disorders around the world. Recent evidence suggests that these treatment effects are overestimated due to several factors, such as publication bias, researcher allegiance, and other shortcomings in study design (Ioannidis, 2005; Ioannidis, 2008; Driessen et al., 2015; Tajika et al., 2015; Cuijpers et al., 2016; Leichsenring et al., 2017; Leucht et al., 2017; Cuijpers et al., 2019; van Os et al., 2019; cited in Leichsenring et al., 2019).

Leichsenring et al.'s (2019) results for the efficacy of psychotherapy and pharmacotherapy are sobering, finding only a small incremental gain over treatment as usual (TAU) or placebo. This limited incremental gain needs to be balanced against the efforts, costs, and side effects associated with psychotherapy and pharmacotherapy. The situation is aggravated by the numerous concerns mentioned such as biases, inflated studies, and stagnating or decreasing effect sizes, raising serious doubts about the available evidence.

The state of care and avalanche of money spent for children and adolescents, in which there remains so much unmet need, is shameful for a country as wealthy as the United States and other developed countries like New Zealand. Reviewing these statistics gave me a profound sense of hopelessness. These brilliant statisticians, leaders in their field, have thrown down the gauntlet challenging our field to change. We are failing our consumers—children, families, the chronically mentally ill, and other troubled people asking for our help. This unmet need is not for lack of trying.

This failure gnawed at me. These daunting, depressing statistics seemed ubiquitous and demanded challenge. Trained by the titans of the field, really smart people who gave me my foundations and brilliant ideas on how to treat patients gave me the knowledge and experience that psychotherapy, especially family therapy, can transform problematic systems. The outrage I felt from deep within is the knowledge that it didn't have to be this way, all this failure. With those trendy treatment models, fashionable and oh so politically correct, smartly dressed, did not live up to their promises. With this, I set about to find a solution; RBA answered the call.

In the middle 1990s, government agencies experienced a dilemma: many programs were claiming to alleviate the problems of children and adolescents, and yet there was little or no data on their effectiveness. Large sums of money were allocated with scant attention to measuring their results. The RBA accountability framework was developed to address this problem. RBA operates at two levels: population accountability and performance accountability. In each case, it provides a disciplined way of thinking and taking action that can produce change.

At the level of population accountability, RBA asks what quality of life conditions do we want for the children, adults, and families who live in our community? These "population results" are intended to take on big matters of wellbeing like a clean environment, a safe community, and physically and mentally healthy children and adults. At the population level, indicators are identified to tell us the extent to which these conditions are being achieved. These become the starting point for developing plans that can produce measurable improvement in quality of life.

At the level of performance accountability, performance measures are identified for programs, including the most important measures addressing customer wellbeing or customer outcomes. The same planning methods can produce measurable progress for the full range of programs and their customers. Overall, RBA is a practical model that organizes large and small systems toward measurable improvement.

In 1995, Mark Friedman, having completed 19 years with Maryland's Department of Human Resources, including six years as chief financial officer, was dismayed at the fact that a vast amount of taxpayers' money and charitable foundations' money was being spent with little to no data on whether these programs were achieving required outcomes. In Friedman's view, agencies typically used an "industrial model" much like a factory. Resources were the input, and the only measurable output was the service delivery itself. In contrast, the RBA model he developed is a change model, guided by questions like: How much service did we provide? How well are our services being delivered? Are we achieving the desired outcomes for our customers? The condensed version of these three categories of performance measurement is spare but complete: How much did we do? How well did we do it? Is anyone better off?

I experienced a similar challenge firsthand, in 1995, when I was the chief medical officer of a Medicaid Behavioral HMO in Philadelphia. The institution was well funded, with an annual budget of millions of dollars, funding a vast array of services. Yet, our system could not find a workable framework to track our providers' outcomes.

While I was leading the clinical program, we recruited national experts to advise on the selection of an outcome system. One of them said all we needed to do was to check whether our clients were satisfied with their treatment. We agreed that client satisfaction was important to consider but not worthy of being the single treatment metric. After all, as we clinicians well know, self-reported satisfaction is a tenuous measurement. Clients' desire to please their therapists, among myriad other factors, ensures that satisfaction does not necessarily correlate with effective treatment outcomes. Furthermore, satisfaction is subjective by definition, certainly not a grounded measure of wellbeing or functionality.

A second expert suggested that we learn from Nike and "just do it." Tracking outcomes is so challenging, he posited, that as long as you are engaging in a credible, tested process, that is sufficient. He seemed to think that the intention was all that mattered. This naivety didn't work for us.

The third expert just told jokes! (More nihilism.) We were looking for an effective framework and clearly, at that point, it appeared tracking outcomes was in the "too hard basket." The solution I ultimately found was RBA.

I attended a leadership development conference held at a Native American reservation on the upper peninsula of Michigan in the mid-1990s. The welcoming words of the tribal elder moved me greatly; the tribe planned for seven generations. Planning like this is, of course, in marked contrast to most Western businesses, which only plan for the next quarter. During the retreat, I learned that this tribe was the first Native American community to introduce gambling in the United States. Years earlier, as the elders were walking by a local church in their impoverished community, they noticed an advertisement for bingo. One had looked to the other and said, "In some way, the church has been able to 'bend the rules' because they are a special population." His compatriot replied, "Hey, we're Indians, we're special too." They embraced the idea of their uniqueness as Native Americans and borrowed the gambling concept and ultimately built a casino. Boy, did that take off. It became a fast-growing source of funding for social services that were available to all members of the tribe. Years later, I continue to be captivated by this small tribe's leadership.

Mark Friedman's RBA model for leaders was the major focus of this conference in Michigan. I was impressed with RBA; it was concise, concrete, and practical. Most striking was its emphasis on measurement and the importance of involving all the stakeholders at the beginning and throughout the initiative's operation. Immediately, I began to speculate further about the model's applicability to family therapy. Its prioritization of the use of low-cost or no-cost resources was something family therapists intuitively understood in their work. There is no lower-cost resource than the family. A major commonality between family therapy and RBA is that both are in the business of changing systems.

RBA is so logical and contrary to the deadening arbitrary administrative "groupthink" of most outcome systems. RBA is committed to the heresy of common sense.

When governments adopted the RBA framework, the administrators were nervous. They watched tentatively as their systems began a transformation. The leaders realized that their large systems were no longer plodding along; elephants were dancing.

Mark Friedman started a revolution. He spent many years beating the bushes, passionately spreading his ideas. I remember him describing near-empty classrooms in small towns in the Mid-West when he first started. And years later, as his revolution gained wide acceptance, he shared a stage in South Korea at the OECD World Forum. RBA now spans at least 15 countries and 50 states. Friedman's book, *Trying Hard Is Not Good Enough*, has sold 70,000 copies and counting (Friedman, 2015). It has been translated, in whole or part, into at least 15 languages including Mandarin.

It was "déjà vu, all over again," as I confronted the same problem in Auckland. As clinical director of this residential program for troubled adolescents, there was no capacity to determine how well we were doing. I contacted Mark Friedman and asked for his collaboration in developing an outcome-tracking system based on our respective models: RBA and IST. We ventured into the unknown and produced a model with the ability to assess potent interventions that could be measured. This simplified system of care was designed to be respectful, pay attention to the complexities, recognize the fragmentation and the ability to reach wide into the community and the bigness of life. Over the 15 years, our staff tweaked, reshaped, and reconfigured components that would sharpen our work with this amalgamated model for front-line clinicians. It just seemed like the obvious solution for the families that so desperately needed our help. We learned and grew, and our outcomes improved. Everyone participated in the success.

The IST/RBA Model

There are nine tenets of the IST/RBA Model; these are described through the process of supervision I was providing to a child psychiatrist. They reflect how the model is conceptualized and delivered.

Case

When COVID struck the world, Auckland shut down. "Go fast and go hard," was the message of the prime minister, a venerable rugby slogan.

Mia and her family were confined together, like millions of others. That's when the assaults began on the 16-year-old Bangladeshi girl. She withdrew, hid in her bedroom, and then in desperation called social services, "Please, take me away, my family is killing me." I was supervising a child psychiatrist who was overseeing her care in a government-funded program.

Mia had been in and out of the medical system for two years with a diagnosis of anorexia nervosa that, at this point, was questionably under control. She is the middle child of three, with an older sister who is 19 and a younger brother of 12. The father is a successful engineer, consulting across many countries, and was rarely home before COVID struck. The mother is a homemaker. The family had lived in England, Melbourne, and now Auckland. They are active in the Muslim community.

Social service supported Mia in a crisis refuge accommodation; a temporary safe-haven, with nurturing staff, while a coordinated plan could be established.

Tenet One: Bring All the Stakeholders Together

The first step in RBA is to bring all the stakeholders together; this is the duty of the therapist. The stakeholders were the family, social service, the pediatrician (because of the anorexia), the school supervisor, a state-appointed lawyer for Mia, the therapists, the general practitioner, and the Imam. The mother and father, although perpetrators of this abuse, must be a part of the plan from the beginning. There was no imperative to emancipate this 16-year-old.

With young Mia teetering on fulminant anorexia and soon to be a run-away on the streets, I told my supervisee that the danger for this teenager was high. I cautioned that every stakeholder must commit to the establishment of an organized system of care. A system is defined as a group of people associated to achieve a common purpose. There was flexibility, of course, to include new stakeholders as they emerged.

The classic book by Donald Berwick et al., *Curing Health Care* (1991), with its opening riveting anecdote, reminds us of the necessity of accountability of collaborators. All stakeholders should be involved with the change agenda creating a collaborative plan of action.

> She died. She didn't have to. The senior resident was sitting near
> tears in the drab office behind the nurses' station in the intensive
> care unit. It was 2 am, and he had been battling for 32 hours to save
> the life of the 23-year-old graduate student who had just suffered
> her fatal cardiac arrest. The resident slid a large manila envelope
> across the desktop. "Take it; look at this." The routine screening
> chest X-ray was taken 10 months ago. The tumor was right there,
> and it was curable—then. By the time the second film was taken
> eight months later, because she complained of pain, it was too
> late, the tumor had spread everywhere, and the odds were hope-
> lessly against her. "Everything we have done since then has really
> just been wishful thinking. We missed our chance. She missed her
> chance." Exhausted, the resident put his head in his hands and
> cried. The young woman's initial X-ray had been misplaced; it slid
> to the floor and was thrown out.

This system, as Berwick described, failed to work as a unit; the many
stakeholders were unaware of each other's responsibility. Was the fatal
flaw with the radiologist who read the X-ray, or the negligence of the
internist who ordered the study and didn't follow-up? Or, as Berwick
asks, "was it the radiology department manager who did not have the
budget that year to purchase an X-ray tracking system? Or the secretary
who was a 'Temp' and did not know the administrative procedures?"
(Berwick et al., 1991, p. 3).

Tenet Two: Agreement on the Outcomes

The stakeholders determine the desired outcomes of treatment, avoiding the fragmentation of services that can undo even the best of plans.
In what way do we want this person/client to be better off? And how
will we know in measurable terms the extent to which we are achieving
these desired conditions? This perspective greatly minimizes an unpro-
ductive, meandering adherence to clinical models and processes.

Everyone, except the parents, agreed that the violence against Mia
must stop. The non-Western culture of this family, living in a developed country for many years, with three teenagers, presented a cultural
clash of immense proportions. Mia's lawyer was firm in her words to the

parents that New Zealand does not tolerate child abuse and warned them that they were at risk of prosecution. The parents acknowledged that the stress in the home, leading to the violence, should be diminished and resolved. They understood and agreed to cooperate. Mia's weight and ameliorating her anorectic symptomatology were prioritized, as was eliminating family violence.

Tenet Three: Agreeing on Data Markers

Friedman says, "Getting professional people to use data to improve performance requires a cultural shift" (Friedman, 2015). Professional stakeholders, with disparate backgrounds, who may not be accustomed to data markers or the scientific orientation of tracking data, present a challenge. They sometimes struggle with understanding that the most important measurements are grounded, objective, observable markers.

A psychoanalytic therapist asked me about one of her clients who was increasingly dysphoric and reclusive. I asked her how long she had been working with her. "Seventeen years," was her reply. There seemed no urgency for change with her model of therapy. More importantly, I could not ascertain any data measures for progression. As clinicians, we are so often enchanted by the process dimension in the treatment room that we ignore asking if anyone is better off.

Mia's visits to the home, from her crisis accommodation, increased; they were agreed measurements and indicated that the home context was becoming more salutary. The biweekly weights of Mia were recorded and reported to the general practitioner. I suggested that the psychiatrist should review the characteristics of a "psychosomatic family" and then organize measuring, especially the degree of triangulation. The conflict avoidance characteristic must be continuously monitored.

Peter Drucker, the father of business journalism, famously wrote, "If you can't measure it, you can't manage it" (Zak, 2013). As therapists, we are managers of the system's change. We track grounded numerical information. The measures are utilized to track progress against a desired goal. In RBA, there is an implicit continuous cycle of review and refinement through this data-driven approach.

Most managers know how the program works. They should be able to identify three to five of the most important measures in their program, explain how the program is doing on these measures and what can be done to improve the program's performance (Friedman, 2015).

One of the important issues, according to Friedman, is picking the right performance measures. He says, "it is a fence drawing problem and first we draw a fence around the thing to be measured. It could be a program, or a component of a program" (Friedman, 2015). Alternatively, I suggest, it could be a youngster's behavior and/or overall functioning, it could be family functioning, or it could be the entire clinical program, i.e., Windsor House.

Tenet Four: Using the Clinical Scorecard

The integration of IST and RBA principles helped create the Clinical Scorecard that measures performance over time. This valuable tool tracked the clinical effectiveness of the episodes of care and informed the team if it was achieving these temporal goals. It did serve as a reveille at times, alerting the stakeholders when markers were askew.

The Scorecard empowered the clinical team via the tracking of pivotal measurable parameters, increasing accountability for progress. Progress toward consensually chosen goals, which were determined at the outset by the therapy team, the family, the client, and other professionals, was tracked continuously via this tool. It supports a timeframe to develop sustained improvement (Table 3.1).

Tenet Five: Plan of Action

A collaborative plan of action is different from the individual plans of the respective professionals. It is not an amalgamation of the plans but an agreed single treatment agenda.

The family therapist leads the transformation of the system. In the case of Mia, addressing the marital split and the ensuing triangulation, characteristic of psychosomatic families, will help to restructure the family toward a more functional state. Concurrently, the family therapist will work closely with the pediatrician. The team notes that Mia's increasing

Table 3.1 Clinical Scorecard for Mia

Desired outcomes	Plans	Measures	Targets	Homeostatic maintainer
1 Mia thriving at home	Family therapy	Home visits for Mia	Number and duration 10% improvement first month	Father
2 Mia thriving at school	Possibly a tutor for Mia	School performance (grades)		
3		Triangulation Scale scores		
4		Conflict avoidance scale scores		
5		Psychological test, utilized to determine Mia's suicidality		
6		Anorexia nervosa parameters: Weight tracked biweekly from the baseline		
7				

willingness to return home (number of home visits) indicated that the system was positively changing; the violence was diminished.

Tenet Six: Targets

Targets serve as desired levels of future achievement, often alerting the treatment team to focus and enhance collaboration. They are specific and measurable and bound by a realistic time-period and based on previous performance. They are typically expressed as, "in x period of time, we want to achieve an y percentage of improvement in a behavior." For example, in two months, there will be a 20% increase in school attendance. Progress is measured by determining whether targets have been met. If used correctly, targets produce realistic behavior improvements.

In Mia's case, the team decided that her home visits in a one-month interval would show a 10% increase; the second month, the targets would be adjusted.

Targets, as described in chapter 8, serve as interim outcome measures. Achieving targets indicates to the team that they are progressing towards the team's agreed upon outcomes.

Tenet Seven: The Homeostatic Maintainer

The HM is an individual(s) or an interactional pattern, that, when the system is perturbed, activates to prevent change, maintaining the status quo.

Mia's father, when challenged by his wife, stormed out of the session, making it impossible at that moment to address and resolve their marital issues. We saw him as the HM: when the team challenged the parents to work together, he stormed out of the room, rather than dealing with the family conflicts, thus maintaining the status quo.

Tenet Eight: Turning the Curve

The RBA tool, Turning the Curve, tracks progress from the baseline and performance over time. A baseline is a starting point on a graph, representing historical data. It serves as a warning of where you are headed if we don't do something more, or different, than what we are doing now. In many clinical situations, the graph indicates that the numbers will stay the same or get worse. (Note that a common mistake, according to Friedman (personal communication), is to forecast where you *want* to go, not where you *are* going if you don't do something more or different.) Progress is defined as turning the curve away from the baseline and toward relevant targets. This sets up the following Turn the Curve thinking process: (1) What is the *story behind the baseline?* This discussion addresses causes and forces at work in the past and in the expected future. All partners contribute to this discussion. (2) Who are all the potential *partners with a role to play* in getting better? This is an opportunity to think creatively about partners who are not actively engaged (e.g., a schoolteacher or extended family member). (3) *What works,* or what could work to do better? This step draws on research about effective methods but is *not* limited to the research. The team can use its deep knowledge of the family and community, and common sense, to consider practical actions that have not been formally studied by research, including no-cost and low-cost ideas. (4) Out of this thinking, options for short-term and longer-term action can be identified and an *Action Plan* created. This thinking process (measurement baseline—story—partners—what works—action) can be repeated in some form at each team meeting. Everyone contributes.

Each client functions as their own control. This tool provides the team with an opportunity to adjust plans and interventions. In mental health, baseline curves present a challenge to the team to strive on the most important measures of child, family, and community wellbeing. It goes beyond the episodes of care to the complete course of treatment. It tells the team if they are headed in the right direction (Figures 3.1–3.3).

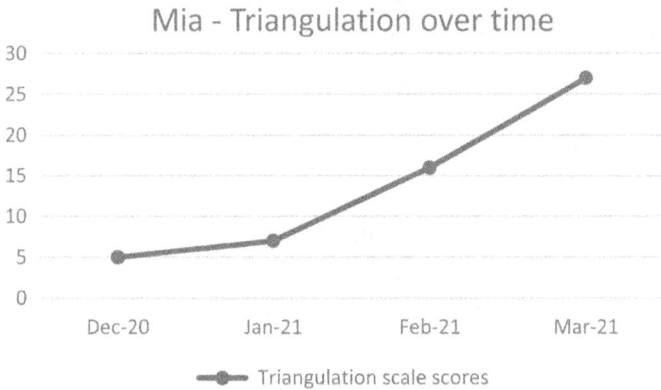

Mia - Triangulation over time

Triangulation scale scores

Figure 3.1 Triangulation Scale scores in Mia's family (a high score indicates less triangulation).

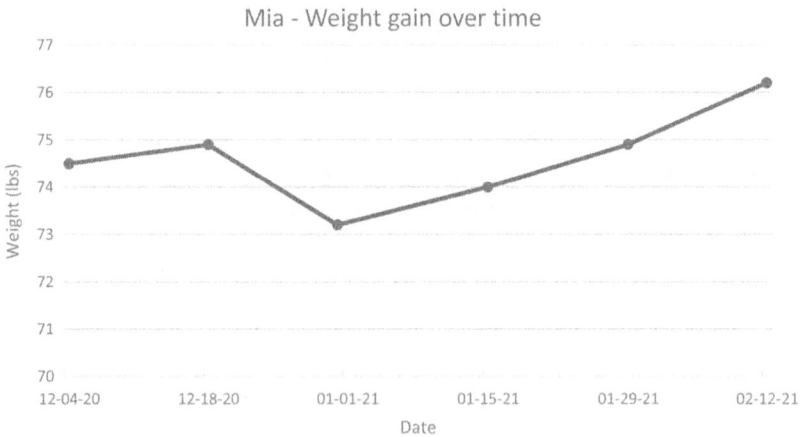

Mia - Weight gain over time

Figure 3.2 Turning the Curve on Mia's anorectic symptoms (weights recorded fortnightly by the clinical team).

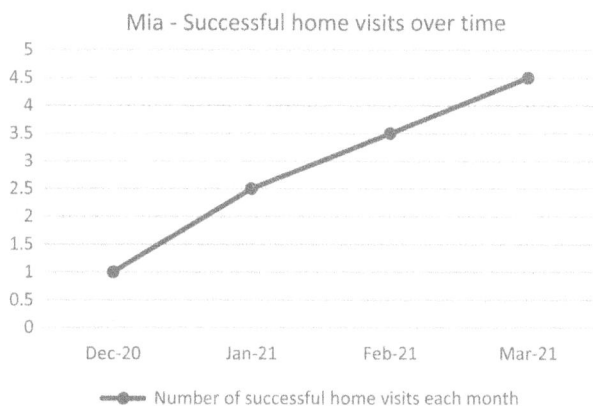

Figure 3.3 Mia's successful home visits.

Tenet Nine: Listening to the Family at Conclusion of Treatment

The phenomenology of the families' experience should be explored; their respected voices may reach far into the future. The treatment team has an opportunity to respectfully accept their feedback. Customer satisfaction informs the system. Freedman recommends a Consumer Feedback Evaluation Tool, deemed "the world's shortest" (see Appendix, page 214). You may adapt the tool to measure satisfaction as required in these areas: What are you doing right; what did you miss; and how you might improve treatment?

Performance Measurement Models

Performance measurement models, known to the field since the 1960s, fail to take the definition of success to the top of the page and use this definition to drive action plans and budgets. RBA breaks from a long-standing tradition of "mission goals" and "objectives" by directly addressing what a client really needs, and what it will look like in measurable terms when they get it (Friedman, 2015). This is a jump in efficiency through grounded performance measures rather than abstract value statements and vague goals relating to clients' wellbeing or satisfaction.

I reviewed many models in the development stage to compare with RBA: the Industrial Model, Change Model, Logic Model, Goal Attainment

Scaling Model, Outcome Funding Framework Model, and the Targeting Outcomes of Programs Model.

The Goal Attainment Scaling Model is a formalized system of tracking goals (Kiresuk & Sherman, 1968) and has many of the same underlying philosophies of the Clinical Scorecard described earlier. It has been validated and shown to have strong reliability. However, the model has been criticized for containing problems about the calculation of standard scores, making it less user-friendly than the RBA model (MacKay et al., 1996).

RBA's simple principles can be applied as easily to the practice of an individual clinician as they can be applied to the functioning of a nationwide health service provider. The use of grounded performance measures as the focal point for performance evaluation, and the attribution of accountability equitably, implicates all involved parties in a system of collective responsibility (Friedman, 2015). The RBA framework is far more versatile and has more significant implications through programs and population initiatives than some previously favored models that focus solely on abstract goal attainment. This is perhaps why it has been adopted by government systems and NGOs around the globe.

The Industrial Model was widely utilized in the private sector, tracking industrial processes by converting raw materials into finished products. However, industrial processes typically do not translate well to private and public sector agencies that provide services to clients or customers. On the assembly line, "materials in, products out" is not valued in human services. Quantity is not the most important type of measure (e.g., the number of psychotherapy sessions). More important are measures of how well we delivered the service. And most importantly of all, the "Is anyone better off?" (customer outcome) measures that help quantify the quality of positive change. I remember asking the general manager at a mental health clinic, "How exactly do you see your job?" She replied, "I see my job as ensuring that all the positions are filled, and that all the workers see their requisite number of clients." Taken aback, I suggested that perhaps the clients would be better served if she tracked their outcomes and analyzed the data toward a values-based approach. That would have required her to change her thinking from the industrial model to an outcome paradigm; this would require a shift in shared responsibility.

According to Friedman, the logic model is one of the most widely utilized frameworks in the United States. Both frameworks are logical—the major difference between RBA and the Logic Model is RBA's focus on measured performance (Friedman, 2015). The logic model believes that there is a continuum between program and population effectiveness.

> A number of other conceptual models, notably those with roots in the logic model literature, tend to reinforce the flawed view of a linear relationship between performance and population accountability. These models do not sharply distinguish between the two. Instead, they often present a smooth continuum from inputs to outputs to outcomes to community results. There is nothing to suggest that crossing over from performance to population conditions is anything more than the next step in this linear progression. The models tend to encourage managers to think they have some form of prime responsibility for the community condition that their program aims to impact. This way of thinking is counterproductive. It heightens fear in managers and takes energy away from their efforts to improve performance. RBA works in the opposite direction from logic models: from community results backward to programs. In this direction, the non-linear relationship is obvious. If we want to measurably improve water quality, then we must consider the potential contributions of many partners with a role to play, not just the Water Quality Division. (Friedman, 2015)

This population-based reality was reinforced to me by the experience of a friend. Bill had sold his business and enrolled in the University of Pennsylvania Teacher's College. He spoke passionately of his vision for teaching adolescents. He had many inventive ideas on how to make a difference in these young lives, like in the classic movie, *Lean on Me*. "Stemming the tide," Bill said, referring to the lost youth in our four-centuries-old city with both beautiful and decrepit neighborhoods. He was on fire, truly inspired.

I bumped into him on the street two years later. I said, "Hey Bill, how's your teaching going?"

> Oh that; I left after six months. It was chaos. The kids were ok in the classroom, but the real cacophony was within the school system and beyond. The teacher fought with the principal, the principal with the commissioner of education, who in turn fought with the mayor. The kids would go home to even more chaos: poverty, drug-laden communities, and, for some of the most star-crossed, HIV.

Looking determinedly, he said, "I'm a stockbroker now." And he went on his way.

There's an old saying: *Serving soup until your elbows fall off is not the way to end hunger!* Bill apparently realized the futility of his quest. There needed to be a concomitant population-based change process; looking at the community and working backward.

In 2008, the city of Leeds, England, failed its government-based Children's Services Audit (Leeds City Council, 2015). The services were deemed sub-standard; there were far too many young people in custody. The city charged its director, Nigel Richardson, to reorganize children's social care.

Using RBA principles, Richardson triggered a shift. This shift went beyond a child-centered orientation to a focus on the family and the community. The "Family Valued" Project mobilized the entire city of Leeds (population approximately 700,000) around implementing a restorative, family-centered model to specific outcomes for its children. The Turning the Curve tool was used to show progress and the city adopted this methodology for many other issues as a city-wide approach. The performance-tracking tool for children showed the four most important measures and became known as a "Thing of Beauty." After four years, Leeds city-wide had turned the curve on all four measures. In this newly organized system of care, the entire community had access to the data, and this allowed them to participate in tracking the outcomes and adjusting plans locally; and they listened and responded to the children (Leeds City Council, 2015).

Figure 3.4 demonstrates that the entire city, even including the park service, was involved in the "Family Valued" project. The "Weekly Obsessions Tracker" data demonstrate both the positive progress and the close tracking of their data, which according to Richardson was widely distributed to stakeholders (personal communication, 2018) (Figure 3.5).

A Casey Foundation colleague, Molly Layton-Tierney, described in her TED talk a population-centered initiative, using the RBA framework. Over five years, she led her team to decrease the number of children in the Baltimore City, Maryland, foster care system by 58%. Her team was

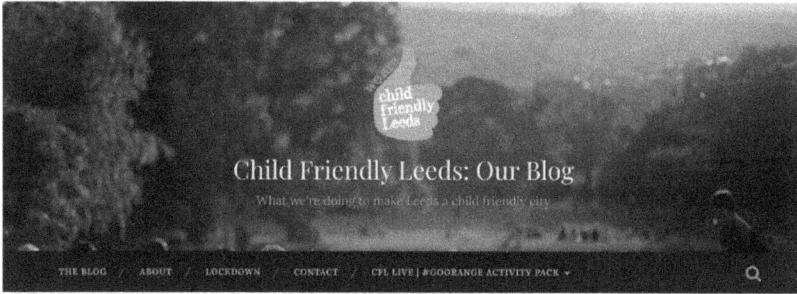

Figure 3.4 Image from the Child Friendly Leeds blog webpage.

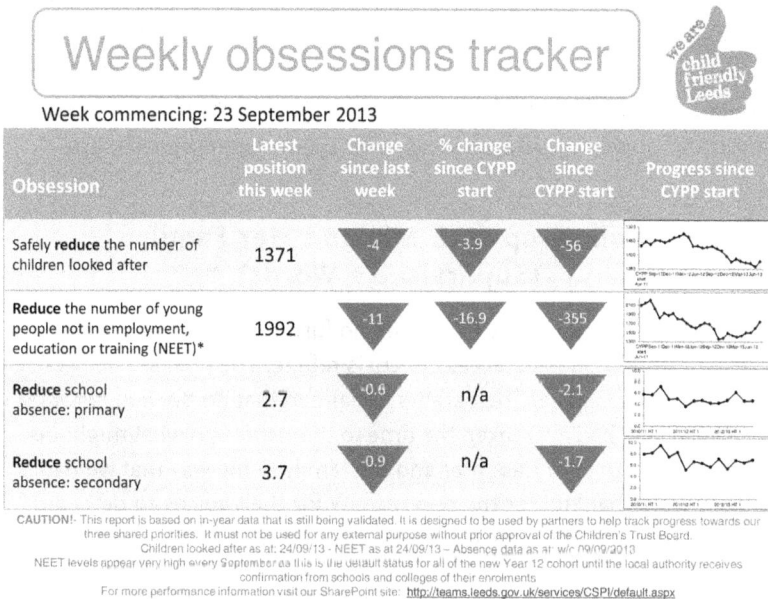

Figure 3.5 Child Friendly Leeds "Weekly obsessions tracker" NEET, not in employment, education, or training.

successful in reducing approximately 89% of children from orphanages, and 59% of children in state custody, and moving 47% from foster care to families (TEDx, 2014). All without an increase in rates of child abuse and neglect (the safety check measure).

Molly organized stakeholders around a single mission and collected data. She combated the lack of coordination by creating an internal organization complete with case management staff, operation staff, personnel staff, caseworkers, financial managers, facility workers, and supply clerks—all with a focus on their agreed-upon outcomes. The purpose of this reorganization was to demonstrate full inclusivity from the outset; the caseworkers who were providing the treatment would be fully supported as "one working system," instead of separate individual parts.

Conclusion

Most family therapists understand that a congruent child and family system needs to be created because too often there can be a blatant lack of coordination. The same certainly applies to large public social systems like Molly Layton-Tierney's in Baltimore, as well as Nigel Richardson, in Leeds, in which they transformed large community children's services using these powerful, simple ideas with their talented leadership.

Follow-up with Mia and Her Family (Supervisee's Words)

Mia is back home. There have been no further violent episodes and she has not requested access to crisis refuge. The final session was remarkably positive. The parents exclaimed that no previous group of clinicians had ever taken the time to think through what might be going on with their daughter and the family in the way that we had. They were thankful for the opportunity for their voices to be heard and the time that we took for them.

4

INTENSIVE STRUCTURAL THERAPY STREAMLINED

Forty years ago, a patient would undergo a lengthy procedure to remove cataracts, including a two-week hospitalization—in bed, with the windows shaded and sandbags on each eye. If they survived this convalescent period, they would tentatively be ready to go home. Today, the patient, fully dressed, walks into the operating room and reclines. The surgeon makes a small incision replacing the patient's lens. This takes less than seven minutes. The patient stands up and walks to the recovery room for cookies and a cup of tea. The next day, when the patch is removed, the patient marvels at the brightness of the room; vision is clear, the world is in Technicolor again! Driving is now safe, with a life transformed.

An effective disruptive force like the surgery above, family therapy, at its inception was revolutionary. And now, decades later, the need for disruption in mental health has never been greater. The troubling statistics about treatments that don't work beg for this change. Treatments must be more effective, faster, more inclusive, more cost-effective, and more

DOI: 10.4324/9781003161257-5

equitable to better serve our clients and families. This chapter offers a modest proposal to reach this goal.

Structural family therapy, the genius of Salvador Minuchin, and a bombshell of disruption when introduced, is the foundation from which I developed my model. The streamlined intensive structural therapy (IST) model presented here has been parsed for what gets the best-measured outcomes, providing a framework to transform the presenting problems. What has been removed are therapeutic elements that do not lead to fast change—or, frankly, change at all.

Conceptualizing the presenting problem acontextually, or not directing treatment toward restructuring the contemporary system, leads often to a clinical cul-de-sac. The key element of system dysfunction is triangulation; it is the schism between the parental figures. "The split" often recruits a third person to come between the couple—usually a child, sometimes a grandmother, or friend. This ubiquitous triangulated structure in the family system keeps the dynamics locked, maintaining the presenting problem. Focusing on triangulation at the start results in the ability to quickly and efficiently simplify the treatment. It is Ariadne's thread that is unrolled to transform the system.

Most frequently in clinical case conferences, the clinician describes an avalanche of patient and family characteristics, often failing to acknowledge the war at the heart of the family—the conflict in the parental unit. In one case, a 15-year-old female was in an inpatient psychiatric unit, anorectic and self-harming; she had been hospitalized previously. Almost off-hand, the psychiatrist mentioned that the parents were "at odds, consistently disagreeing on issues concerning their daughter." Off-hand will not get to the heart of the problem but will likely lead to repeated hospitalizations for this 15-year-old.

The HM concept compliments the therapy. It is the clinical "searchlight" informing who keeps the system "stuck" and offers quick direction to the therapist. It creates focus and intensity and gives the clinician a potent point of incisive intervention. A commercial on TV many years ago, when a woman picks up a hamburger and says, "Where's the beef?", took the country by storm in its pointed simplicity. The correct lens for the family therapist at the start will lead the clinician to "the beef"—the HM.

One of the significant advantages of this treatment model is the ease of tracking family processes in the therapy room; the trained eye observes the changes in the structural patterns in real time. Patients are not sent home to practice or work on their issues. Their dynamic patterns are transformed here and now. When teaching, Salvador Minuchin frequently referred to this interactional process as the "family dance" (personal communication, 1974). This dance, this flow of interactions, is rarely consciously manifested. In polite society, of course, we are trained to edit our words, but not our unconscious transactional processes which, ever apparent to trained observers, are rarely self-censored by the uninitiated.

What follows is the core curriculum of IST, shaped through treating and supervising an immeasurable number of cases. The following concepts together will transform systems.

Concept One: "Everything is Connected"

Thinking in Systems, authored by Donella Meadows (2008), states that a system isn't just any old collection of things. A system is an interconnected set of elements that is coherently organized in a way that achieves something (Meadows, 2008). These constituent parts interrelate over time, within the context of larger systems. Of course, this is the basis of the family therapy paradigm.

With troubled young people, therapists frequently must work at the edges of the clients' family system, doing their best to include everyone who is influential. In the Windsor House program, the vast majority of the clients belonged to complicated, often large, impoverished, multicrisis families. Substance abuse ran rampant both in the parental generation and with the adolescents. There was often a complexity of relationships with stakeholders—schools, courts, the police, and peers of the young people. Their participation in the treatment was vital. Social Services were charged by the court to keep the youngsters in a safe place, and paid Windsor House, the in loco parentis custodians, to find a solution for the problematic, often dangerous behaviors. Such a daunting complexity of systems mandates the inclusion of all influential stakeholders.

Concept Two: The Extracorporeal Mind

Underpinning IST is the theory of the mind in context; the extracorporeal mind. Gregory Bateson espoused that the mind is immanent in one's social context (Bateson, 2002). Our consciousness is populated by our day-to-day relationships. In this theory, the clinician diligently searches for those current relationships that lead to the expression of the presenting problem/s and becomes the venue for the amelioration of the symptoms. The cause of the problem is lost in history, not directly knowable. Notable exceptions are posttraumatic stress disorder (PTSD) and similar conditions where the past may actively intrude on consciousness and contribute to symptom expression.

If one speculates on the process of evolution, our progenitors did not evolve by contemplating their childhoods. Instead, our evolutionary forebears (to whom we owe much gratitude, thank you) were in constant danger. They were focused on survival. They were busy looking over their shoulders, to stay alive. Leaving, frankly, little time for introspection. That is the here and now—the contemporary context.

This paradigm goes beyond the constraint of the "self" by historical determinants, and instead focuses on the contemporary interactions with the environment and significant others; the "extracorporeal mind." In fact, the context triggers certain characteristics within the individual, causing other characteristics to become unattended and psychologically unimportant. Depending on the demand characteristics of the context, certain facets prevail, while less functional facets recede. It is a figure-ground shift. Therefore, the individual's social ecology calls forth the more functional facets of personality. As a result, this concept encompasses the "self" in context—the mind is a "changeable," responding entity. Indeed, our conscious minds are ever checking our context for information and feedback.

The more a clinician maintains fealty to the Batesonian concept of mind in context, and clarity of purpose is established, the more successful is the treatment. It is not necessary to capitulate to the current fashion in psychotherapy that imposes pressure to incorporate other therapy models for therapeutic integration. On the contrary, to do so would confound attempts toward proof of concept. Determining an effective therapeutic model would be difficult if they were all squashed together. I stick with the Batesonian concept.

In writing a paper, "The Psychosomatic Family in Child Psychiatry," with Salvador Minuchin (Minuchin & Fishman, 1979), we used Bateson's metaphor to clarify the family-oriented practitioner's concept of "self." Bateson described a blind man walking down the street with a cane in his book, *Steps to an Ecology of Mind* (Bateson, 1972). Several hypothetical questions emerged: Does the "self" of the blind man end at the hand holding the cane? Does his "mind" include the cane down to its end, but before it touches the sidewalk? Or, should we consider that his "mind" ends in the middle of the cane? This example presents a way of conceptualizing the individual so that the "mind" includes the feedback from the blind man's context. From this perspective, the "mind," or "self," at a given moment, is the result of a person's previous experiences, their biology plus the dominant characteristics of their social context.

Recent theories about social networks have provided supporting data for Gregory Bateson's concept. Influential moods can be contagious, according to Bond's research on social networks. This social contagion can affect an individual's level of happiness and depression, as well as behaviors like drinking, smoking, and eating habits (Bond, 2014).

Harvard psychiatrist, and sociologist, Nicholas A. Christakis, and UC San Diego professor of political science and medicine, James H. Fowler, have advanced our understanding of social networks (Fowler & Christakis, 2008). They analyzed the longitudinal data from the Framingham Heart Study, a long-term, ongoing, cardiovascular cohort on residents of the town of Framingham, Massachusetts. The study began in 1948 with 5,209 adult subjects from Framingham and in 2002 commenced working with its third generation of participants. Their focus was on the social networks including spouses, caregiving relationships, neighbors, and other social connections. Fowler and Christakis explored factors such as the spread of network health behaviors (e.g., obesity) and other network health-related phenomena (e.g., depression and death). Twelve thousand people (including family, friends, and neighbors) were followed for over 30 years. Results indicated that both weight gain and weight loss appeared to extend along with social network ties.

Importantly, results from this famous study showed that happy people within close geographic proximity are most effective in transferring their good cheer (happiness) to others and that the most satisfied people are the ones at the center of large social networks. Fowler and Christakis found that happiness increases among friends and family. Therefore, a happy friend who lives within a half-mile of you can, and often will, make you happy. Moreover, you have a 42% chance of becoming happier after speaking to or spending time with a friend or relative who is happy. However, if the friend or relative lives approximately two miles away, this impact drops to 22%. Likewise, you are 14% more likely to be happy if you have happy siblings; however, this only applies if you live within one mile of each other. Similarly, Dr. Peter Totterdell, a psychology research fellow at The University of Sheffield, found a link between happiness in professional cricketers during a match, and the happiness of nurses during their shift work (Bond, 2014). From my perspective, this research is sociological confirmation of the mind in context theory. The "self" is profoundly influenced by and, indeed, extends to the social context.

Concept Three: Theory of Change—Establish Congruence to Build an Organized System of Care

A theory of change underlies clinical models. With CBT, "Change cognitions and emotions are modified"; with psychopharmacology, emotional change results from modifications in brain chemistry. IST posits that clinical change occurs when the clinician establishes a congruent, organized system—all the stakeholders "speaking with one voice." In my experience with young people, there are rarely organic causes to explain their presenting emotional or behavioral problems. Rather, their social context, usually their family system, is creating the stress leading to the dysfunction. When a system is rendered congruent, the client's problems and symptoms mitigate. The need for a coherent context applies universally and the chronically mentally ill have benefited from this concept. The documented effectiveness of family psychoeducation, creating an organized system, moderates psychotic symptomatology by reducing the level of expressed emotions (EE) within the family and changing the degree of family discord (Lincoln et al., 2007).

In my teaching, I use the metaphor of a clock to graphically demonstrate this "theory of change." A clock fails if all the parts do not smoothly coordinate. If a mechanism is stuck, you'll be late for your meeting. Clinically, when there is a discordance in the therapeutic system, there is an increased probability that behavioral or psychiatric symptoms will exacerbate.

Each clinician has an obligation to investigate: Are there members of the therapeutic system who are not working together? Where is the split in the system? Is the social worker collaborating? Have you joined with the family? Are the father and mother sabotaging each other? Find areas where congruence can be repaired.

Concept Four: The Multifaceted "Self"

Aware of self-fulfilling prophecies, it is essential for the therapist to believe that their client can manifest more functional aspects of the self. I co-authored a paper about families with disabled children who accept their child's limitations without gentle challenges to do more, and thus the young person does not stretch to grow. To the extent that the child does not push himself, it confirms the family's reality that he is limited. The family and child settle into a mindset of acceptance and the child's capacities remain static (Fishman et al., 1977).

There is a risk of focusing on pathological characteristics manifested by presenting problem/s, and sometimes neglecting the rich repertories that are potentially available to people. Those coping behaviors that have remained dormant as a result of their social context can be awakened. The search for strength is a figure-ground transformation; the dormant parts of the self are brought forth, while others recede. Crucially, this new context maintains these newly expressed, positive aspects.

We must make a distinction between personality and the presenting symptoms. The multifaceted "self" is the complex repertories of thoughts, feelings, and behaviors that represent the individual. Personality, defined as the combination of characteristics or qualities that form an individual's distinctive character, is the composite of genes, experiences, culture, and much more. In our work with the client's contemporary context, we address the system responsible for the maintenance of the presenting problem, not the personality.

Concept Five: Assessing the System

Professor Occam's theory, also known as the "law of parsimony," is a philosophical tool for "shaving off" unlikely explanations. Essentially, when faced with competing explanations for the same phenomenon, the simplest is likely the correct one. Despite his untimely death in 1412, he remains my inspiration and guide (I still miss him).

What follows, in the Occam traditions, is a simple and practical approach to assessment. I offer The One-Minute Assessment Tool for family systems (OMAT) in the same spirit of brevity. It was inspired by the classic book, *The One-Minute Manager* (Blanchard, 2003), which prioritized for its readers the most effective management techniques; it included the wheat, not the chaff. Using the OMAT, you can read structure, identify developmental stages, recruit relevant history, observe the process, and identify the homeostatic maintainer.

Appraise the *family structure* to locate the structural flaws, giving an operational working hypothesis. This is akin to conducting a biopsy of the system. This dynamic lens allows the practitioner to assess and reassess after interventions. You should see the family patterns changing before your eyes, and the presenting problems ameliorating. These quick snapshots do not intend a fixed evaluation that has finality.

Many years ago, I asked Salvador Minuchin how he came upon the idea of structure.

> I was influenced by medicine; I was looking for something similar to the structure of a body organ, like the heart, something with perceivable architecture. From the beginning, I acknowledged that structures are ever-changing. The architectural structures of family systems bend, twist, rotate, and give sway to an invaluable lens into their inner workings.
>
> (Personal communication, 1995)

When watching a video with the sound muted, the mother is on a sofa and her daughters, ages six and four, are playing on the floor. When the father enters the room, the spouses glare at one other and soon appear to be shouting at each other. You note that the girls quickly leave the floor to sit on either side of their mother and embrace her. The therapist, viewing the video, immediately understands the family structure and what needs to change. Structure is the efficient, concise, and undeniable lens.

Structural determination is not a value judgment. One is not prescribing how families should live and behave. It is only relevant when people are seeking relief from their psychological pain that the clinician assesses the system's organization. Again, structural dysfunction is a sign that the family system is not congruent.

Salvador Minuchin said:

> I was always interested in context. In Israel, one day, I was watching some children playing on a beach. There were European, South American youngsters alongside Turkish children. I was struck by the fact that the differences in their cultural contexts were vast, yet there were so many similarities in their family interactional patterns. (Personal communication, 1990)

I often muse to my students that one of the great moments in family therapy history was an American football game in 1955—Army vs. Navy. In that game, instant replay videotaping was first introduced. The introduction of video proved to be a great boon to our young family therapy field. Reviewing videotapes, "instant replays," provided a new lens to detect repetitive sequences. They were able to decipher within these patterns the associations between events, such as perceiving the emergence of symptoms when the parents began to fight. They postulated, by extrapolation, that the symptom served a function in the family. To the degree that the emergence of the symptom diffused the conflict, the family was visibly stabilized. Videotape analysis, a new domain of inquiry, was introduced. The early family therapists, Salvador Minuchin, Braulio Montalvo, and others, would review the interactions by videotape, and provide an entirely new clinical universe of invaluable, grounded information and pedagogy.

Structural considerations for the therapist concern the organization and demarcation of the therapeutic system, the influential relationships in the family and broader system. The therapist must punctuate who should be included in the treatment. And then hypothesize, with an open mind, when a therapeutic impasse arises. Who might be missing?

Families seek therapy most frequently when there are *developmental* passages destabilizing their family system. These events create stress to which family systems react in different ways. Some systems accommodated the changes by transforming the interactional rules under which they operated, thereby allowing new, more functional behaviors. In others, they do not change structural rules; this creates increased stress, often leading to medical or psychological symptoms.

The importance of recognizing *developmental stages* informs the therapist. As therapists, we are aware of individual life cycles and look for the classic transitional stages of children into adolescence, leaving home, courtship, marriage, and procreating. We must also factor in those specific points of adult development that are likely to occur within this classic life cycle: the midlife crisis, the "sandwich generation," retirement, and old age are examples.

The intersection of individual child developmental stages coinciding with individual adult developmental stages creates the necessity for the family system itself to enter into a new organization. This can be a triple-locked door: the father was passed over for promotion, the 14-year-old is blasting demands, while in transition, and the family is faced with changing shape to meet the emerging demands of its family members. When a family system does not accommodate to its new reality, symptoms will be expressed. The therapist must be cognizant of these three developmental domains that will require different structural configurations in proximity and distance.

Critical events force the family system to similarly reconfigure. The death of a child, a house fire, divorce, or a lottery win can throw families into a dissipative state, sometimes suddenly, and create intense stress as the old patterns of interaction no longer fit. This is a tsunami, requiring immense supports to stabilize the hopefully temporarily wobbly family system. It is superimposed on a developing family and the therapist will help to negotiate the developmental undertow.

The history of the system may contribute essential information regarding options to the therapy. We should keep in mind, however, that the history that a family reports reflects only a partial reality, a selective chronicle of screen memories. Families scan their collective reflections, remembering and re-telling what they are concerned about at present. The steps the family has taken to attempt resolution, and the involvement of any other therapists, past and present, may be helpful. Medical diagnoses and medical concerns must be surveyed. Critical events can be relevant.

The solution of a family's suffering is most frequently in their contemporary context, not deeply embedded in historical events. The OMAT removes the unnecessary elaborate history-taking that will distract the therapist and the family. History should be acknowledged, and the clinician should bear witness, but the active ingredient in change is transforming the "here and now" relationships.

Process is the flow of interactions within the system. The observable transformations of members of a system "being" with one another.

It is useful to keep in mind the obvious understanding that descriptions of a system by family therapists are different from those done by anthropologists or novelists. Unlike these colleagues, family clinicians do not maintain a fixed distance from the family. At times, the therapist may become "part" of the system through techniques such as "Joining" and/or "Unbalancing," where the therapist acts as a protagonist in the family drama. Or the therapist can be an observer, operating at "35,000 feet." There is an in and out—or somewhere in between. Regardless of the position, the clinician maintains rapport through confirmation and warmth.

The transactional patterns observed by the therapist are objective, grounded observations in contrast to those reactions that the therapist experiences, which are usually subjective. Therapists may bring into the treatment room many subjective factors that can affect the assessment of family systems. Yellow caution lights should blink if the clinician is working with a difficult adolescent and has a "monster" at home. Resisting the pressures of their personal context should be acknowledged; the therapist must recognize that, to some extent, one's reactions will be affected by professional and personal contexts.

The therapist may become inducted into the interactional culture of the family, and inadvertently assimilate into the family's sequences, thereby losing perspective and objectivity. When all the members of the system are operating in a symmetrical manner and the therapist finds him/herself joining the pattern of anger by arguing, then induction is apparent.

Concept Six: The Homeostatic Maintainer

The term *homeostatic maintainer* denotes the individuals or social forces that activate to maintain the status quo when the system is perturbed, thus maintaining the systemic problem. This concept is one of the most useful assessment techniques available to the family therapist.

The term derives from the word homeostasis, meaning "maintaining the same state." In biology or physiology, homeostasis is a process of maintaining sameness by restoring a system to a state from which it periodically departs. A classic example of a homeostatic mechanism is the thermotactic system in the human body. This system acts as a regulator to maintain body heat at a constant temperature to maximize efficiency both in cell reproduction and in interaction with the environment. As we know, however, there are times of crisis, such as infection or injury, when the critical function of the thermotactic system is to raise body temperature. During these periods, increased temperatures act to enhance the production of white blood cells and destroy infecting agents. While the overall goal of the higher temperature is to improve bodily protection, if this excess heat is maintained for too long a period—if it becomes a new status quo—there can be deleterious side effects.

With a family in crisis, there can be forces at work that act to maintain the status quo in a way that is detrimental to the system by keeping the system from changing in the face of developmental pressures. The HM can be an individual or an interactive process such as conflict avoidance that blocks change. The goal is to determine the origin of the "blockage." The HM works to keep the system "stuck" or in the status quo.

If you use this lens to understand and assess the family system, the HM is easily identified and the dysfunction of the system is as clear as day. A mother described how dangerous her 16-year-old son's behavior was, stealing motorcycles and driving them in neighboring farmers' paddocks. He had been skipping school regularly for this activity, and his father, with a broad smile on his face, said, "Boys will be boys." The smile was the equivalent of winking to his son. The father was not supporting his wife and ignored the potential danger that the mother described. He condoned their son's behavior; the father was the HM.

The algorithm for the homeostatic maintainer can be found in the Appendix.

Concept Seven: Ubiquitous triangles

The focus on triangles has been pivotal from the very beginnings of family therapy. Murray Bowen, Don Jackson, and Mara Selvini Palazzoli all discussed the centrality of triangles in troubled families. Evolutionarily, triangles and triangulation are valuable in stabilizing systems; the presence of a third person can stabilize the system.

I have often speculated that in nature, triangles are a stable structure. The famous architect, Frank Lloyd Wright, designed a mile-high building for Chicago that was a tripod structure. He is quoted as saying that his fascination with geometric shapes started with his interest in the Froebel blocks he played with as a child. These shapes, especially triangles, dominated his architectural practice.

The heart of darkness in the struggle of the family is triangulation. Locating this pattern is sometimes quite easy, other times can be challenging. Solving the geometrical puzzle can determine the transformative course. I remember in my training when Jay Haley said, "You know, how you address a family depends on how you think of the problem" (personal communication, 1974). Do you think of the problem as a problem of one? A problem of two? Or do you see it as a problem of three? The more you see the system as a problem of three, the more likely you are to help the family.

Case One: Ruth

I meet regularly with my child psychiatry colleagues, taking turns presenting cases. Ruth, age 17, was popular, had a high academic ranking, and was active in school sports. Abruptly, at the age of 17, she started withdrawing and became selectively mute. She refused to speak at home. Subsequently, the clinician, who had no family therapy training, discussed the distress in the marriage and the extended family. The clinician focused on the young girl, beseeching her to speak, but was unsuccessful. Eventually, the teen was placed in a psychiatric hospital, where she slowly began to utter a few words to the staff, yet she remained mute with her family.

As I listened to the case, I was concerned. It seemed so apparent—a "failure to launch." This young woman functioned very well everywhere, except at home. Developmentally ready to separate from her family, she became symptomatic. The differential diagnosis for sudden onset of psychiatric symptoms at Ruth's age would include schizophrenia. But that would be manifested outside of the home as well. I've seen this launching pattern many times. This older adolescent girl, ready to differentiate from her family, and symptoms mysteriously appear. I speculated that the family was not ready to let her go. When I related my ideas to my peers, there was an uneasy silence. I went on to suggest that the split between the parents was probably maintaining the symptom and the girl was in a triangulated position. The parental system needed her at home as a stabilizing third.

Case Two: Alice

A 15-year-old anorectic girl from an Asian immigrant family, who steadfastly refused to eat and was severely depressed, had hardworking parents who had discord between them. The inpatient program director advocated electroshock treatment to reduce the teenager's depressive symptoms. I was stunned, and I challenged the decision. "This is likely a family problem and should be addressed first before you consider a treatment that is so invasive." Once again, the heart of the problem was the marital split, which desperately needed to be addressed. We know from the psychosomatic research that these families have triangulation, overprotectiveness, rigidity, and conflict avoidance. Electroshock treatment would not address the parental strife.

Case Three: Natalie

A child psychiatry fellow requested a consultation on a family with whom he had been struggling. After a lengthy discussion with me about the family, we interviewed them together. A two-doctor family with three children—Natalie, a 16-year-old adopted daughter was out of control. There were two younger biological children in the home.

I began the consultation session by asking about the problem. The father, a surgeon, an imposing figure, was the apparent leader of the family. He said to me, "I don't know who to agree with—my daughter or my wife." That was all I needed to hear to make a preliminary assessment—the 16-year-old girl was "impossible" because of the triangulating influence. The father was her ally against her mother. And, although there should have been a generational hierarchy (with the parents together), there wasn't one.

Concept Eight: Results-Based Accountability

The essentiality of a viable framework to measure outcomes has become increasingly more pressing as the medical and psychological world has rightfully embraced quality improvement and accountability. Patients and their families should be confident that the clinical model that is guiding their care is based on grounded data that has been measured against baselines. The patient needs to know that when they start a treatment, there is a skilled therapist, committed to tracking outcomes.

Using RBA, every clinician may readily practice as a "local clinical scientist"; always measuring their outcomes and systemically documenting and analyzing their data to ensure patients that they are striving to become a master therapist. Their scientific approach allows them to practice ethically; their interventions are based on what works.

Of course, RBA is more than a performance measurement platform, it is a systems reform tool. Used well, it facilitates an organization of the system, whether utilized for a program or as a population intervention. The very discipline of focusing on outcomes galvanizes the stakeholders.

Concept Nine: Interventions—Family Therapy Techniques to Transform the System

My therapy is based on the book *Family Therapy Techniques* that I co-authored with Salvador Minuchin many years ago (Minuchin & Fishman, 1981).

Time-honored, these techniques address the deep structures of family systems. The family in front of you with multiple members, most suffering in some way; what do you do in the therapy room? Your role is to find the technique that will help unlock the dysfunction and create change in front of you. The clinician readies him/herself as an agent of change by having a repertoire of techniques; those units of intervention that will have enough valence to create the change. The therapist should use whatever technique is necessary to jar the family from their homeostasis and shift them into a more functional system. Techniques like Joining, Intensity, and Unbalancing become central skills to liberate the families.

This inventory of interventions, called the "Alphabet of Skills Worksheet," is located in the Appendix.

Conclusion

A family doctor in San Francisco complained to her mother, "You know, the children I treat have medical problems. But, my medicine doesn't stem the families' other true ailment, the war between the parents."

5

INTEGRATING RBA AND IST

I arrived at Windsor House, a residential program for severely delinquent youth, and to my dismay, I was faced with a time capsule. The organization had been founded 30 years earlier and nothing had changed. It was in an antiquated, decaying, former camp, located on 40 acres in a suburb. Like their institutional forebears, the children slept in steep bunk beds in cheerless houses.

The clinical program was similarly impervious to the passage of time. It was a medley of psychoanalytic psychotherapy and sand trays, with a hit-or-miss token economy. There were no teams. Indeed, therapists were sole agents, and proud of it.

Most troubling, families were strangers to the program. Social services referred youngsters at the point in which their communities had had enough. The second high-speed midnight chase in a stolen car ensured banishment. Visits home were few. Discharged after a year, the youngster was trundled off to an unchanged and surprised family—"What, they didn't fix him?" The household pressure cooker that had led to the

DOI: 10.4324/9781003161257-6

incarceration remained tense. More worrying, the program seemed to have no inkling that the family was the resource for healing their troubled child. This was a lost opportunity.

In those early days, introducing family therapy was a vexing task. The passivity of the staff, their resounding silence when confronted by innovative concepts, left me feeling empty. In my new country, with its British politeness, it was difficult. I found myself thinking, "Please, break the silence, just disagree with me." I suspected that these ideas made little sense to the staff at this time; their New Zealand training had not included family therapy.

I pushed on. I realized that my words were not enough, and they needed to witness systems in action. I had a videotape, made years earlier by a junior therapist, that I thought might serve to pique their interest in the family as a system and they could appreciate for the first time the circularity of family processes. This, I hoped, would be a pivotal point in their family therapy training. In the video, the parents are in the therapy room with two little children, ages three and six. The six-year-old screamed each time the father began to talk. He was a serious, hulk of a man, and visibly exasperated by this provocation. Violence was in the air. With each needling, the three-year-old would run to the father and grab his hands. He would pick her up onto his lap. At one point, the little girl, feeling less worried when the father reassured the therapist that he did not spank the children, announced that she needed to go to the bathroom. The mother stood and took her hand. The older sister again started screaming, and now the younger child was not available to distract the father and protect her sister. Suddenly, he reached out and pushed her small, six-year-old body off the chair. At this moment in time, the family's well-scripted choreography was dramatically demonstrated. Observable tension within the family, a six-year-old diffusing the angry parental dyad by screaming; a three-year-old protecting her sister from their father, and the mother silently withdrawn. Each member had a role that maintained the status quo, until it didn't.

The staff remained placid. Maybe it was my over enthusiasm or perhaps the ideas were so foreign, but there was little response. I know that the people cross the bar, if you will, to embrace these ideas when they see its power in action.

The real turning point for the clinical staff happened in my supervision of one of the therapists working with a recalcitrant 13-year-old girl refusing to attend school. The therapist had spent many hours trying to cajole this stubborn youngster to no avail. The parents, geographically distant, were flown in to support the child going to school that day; they worked together, under my supervision. It was dramatic. The resistant girl willingly attended and continued her attendance, as the therapist worked on a "speakerphone" with the newly formed parental unit thereafter.

From the perspective of our clinicians, in the beginning, the problem was in the child—"Why in the world does the family have to change?" When the power of the parental intervention was demonstrated, and the 13-year-old went to school, the therapist said, "You know, Charles, this stuff works." How amazed she was that this reasonably simple family intervention could create such a dramatic change. I have seen this often, the family therapy paradigm, when demonstrated, changes hearts and minds. The therapist's enthusiasm infected the others; they became active participants in learning this new model.

The giant NZ social services agency referred these young people to Windsor House; each child had a representative social worker from the agency. They were committed professionals with minimal training in family therapy. They were saddled with mountainous caseloads; overwhelmed, they were understandably anxious, like the parents, for us to "just fix the kids." We needed their support to help locate families and recruit the estranged members. Appreciating their limitations, we turned to the supervisors of these overworked, front-line professionals; they were more available and they had access and knowledge of extended family members, as well as resources to recruit them. Developing relationships higher up in the bureaucracy was the way forward. They would become willing partners in our quest to establish organized systems of care focused on families.

A new culture, with inevitable growing pains, was starting to take hold. Going from a single client, needing to be changed, to accepting a systems paradigm, was gratifying. Then, I dared to introduce RBA. A new universe, tackling grounded data, with the mantra of *measure, measure, measure*; there was skepticism. I was convinced that the staff could incorporate both models and easily appreciate RBA's focus on outcomes. In the past, working with an individual paradigm, the outcome was often disappointing; the young person would re-offend and be returned to us. This sobering reality of the frequent recidivism created an opening for the staff to embrace a new way of working.

Our goal was to improve the life chances for the next generation by mobilizing collective effort around a common vision. In the scientific tradition, the promise of this book is to give you, the reader, facile and effective tools, to promote excellent outcomes. Each model, IST and RBA, has a clear lens and techniques that complement each other. RBA starts with the desired outcome and plans backward from there. IST assesses and transforms systems on the basis of structure and the homeostatic maintainer.

While the initiation of family therapy was ticking along at Windsor House, the introduction of RBA required the clinicians to think differently. In government contexts, according to Mark Friedman, "We must first acknowledge that getting people to use data to improve performance is a culture change; performance accountability should be part of a larger working organizational development to create a healthy and effective workplace" (Friedman, 2015). In our field, many clinicians were trained to focus on the processes of their therapeutic models, assuming, all along, that these practices worked. Clinicians appeared to unquestionably follow the lead and wisdom of their teachers. Tracking outcomes, personally checking whether their treatment had been effective, was rare. Often, there was little accounting for the final result of their clinical input.

The Seven Questions

RBA's Seven Questions for Performance Accountability, Friedman's protocols, were introduced to our clinicians. We used this "Seven Question" framework as an exercise in further developing their understanding of our integrated IST/RBA model. Friedman's Questions were designed for governmental agencies, and Windsor House was a non-governmental mental health service, and the Questions did require some adjustments to accommodate the difference. Nonetheless, they were valuable and instructive.

Question One: Who Are Our Clients?

The New Zealand courts would refer children and families to the New Zealand social services, who, in turn, would delegate the care and treatment to Windsor House. From that perspective, the children and families were our clients.

Question Two: How Do We Measure If Our Clients Are Better Off?

It was not enough to say, "She is feeling better," or "He's behaving better"; this was the old-fashioned method of defining outcomes from the previous program. A numerical scale is required for measuring progress. We chose The Child and Family Functional Assessment Scale (CAFAS; Hodges & Kim, 2000) because it closely aligned with our key value on observable data. It is a robust psychometrically sound instrument designed for five- to 19-year-olds. It tracks eight domains of functioning. Additional tools to gauge progress against baseline measurements and benchmarks were sourced and/or developed.

Question Three: How Do We Measure the Progress of the Treatment?

The Clinical Scorecard was developed to measure the overall progress of each client. The Turning the Curve tool would be applied, every three months. The composite of the curves for all children in the program would be analyzed at 3-monthly intervals. Predictive tools, the Triangulation Scale and Single Parent's Scale, would be applied to predict functioning post-discharge. Follow-up methodologies were required at three months and beyond.

Satisfaction surveys would demonstrate that our consumers—families, referrers, and young people—were satisfied with our service. While this information would not be specific and consumer satisfaction is not an outcome, it is still an important quality parameter. A cost/benefit matrix could be analyzed for the treatment from admission to discharge, arriving to the program, and returning to their family and community. Staff turnover should be tracked for programmatic continuity.

Question Four: How Are We Doing on the Most Important of These Measures?

We discussed with the staff the importance of follow-up. This outcome data, post-discharge, would be critical in measuring success—the effectiveness of our program. We were aware that this would prove to be a challenge. Locating the families, who themselves relocate often, and the social services' rudimentary information technology system, would add frustration and make the task nearly impossible. We knew their social worker turnover was high and therefore the institutional memory would be absent to offer help. The cooperation from the NZ social services, in this area, was expected to be minimal, based on previous experience; tremendous pressures were impacting the national agency at that time.

Question Five: Who Are Our Partners Who Have a Role to Play in Achieving Successful Outcomes?

To provide an organized system of care, building a therapeutic community is essential. Our partners would be those professionals from agencies and institutions that interface with the young person and their family. Schools, churches, and the health care system are important partners in supporting positive change. Counsel for child lawyers, sometimes mentors, and family friends become partners. Work and Income New Zealand, the government agency that provides financial benefits, paying for food on the table—all depend on programs like ours to be successful. The police, ever faithful, play an important role. And very importantly, the wide extended family—aunties and uncles and cousins, and the "grans." Of course, the nuclear family system, the most influential in the child's life, was our critically important partner.

Question Six: What Additional Resources, Including No Cost and Low Cost, Might Be Considered?

We were aware that housing insecurity had increased the overall stress among the families, and, at times, delayed discharge. Housing New Zealand, the agency overseeing access and support, would be an important resource to help solve these problems. Agencies that might help deliver these families from poverty could greatly stabilize the children. Education and job/vocational development opportunities should be investigated. Continuous quality education for the students was not available and huge efforts should be exerted to find a solution to this most basic need. A charter school, having won many awards for its innovative educational approaches, had a keen interest in working with our youngsters who have mammoth educational gaps. A rock school partnership could be developed to stimulate musical interest and enhance talent in many of the youngsters.

Question Seven: What Do We Propose to Do?

We propose to integrate IST and RBA into a model that leads to excellent outcomes. The ideas stimulated from this exercise will help prepare the staff for this new way of working. This will imbue the organization's new culture with a modus operandi. These ideas will guide Windsor House into the future.

With open minds, work began. The new accountability loomed large as we learned along the way. The team pulled together around clear goals for the first time. Old traditional practices would surprisingly pop up, but tedious reminders helped to shape the new culture. The CEO, new to the organization as I was, supported the work. This was refreshing and important. The programmatic integration started to take shape, and measurements and targets were improving. Each new case took us further into the model and reinforced the need for robust discussion and cooperation. What follows are a number of cases, demonstrating our programmatic integration of IST/RBA at Windsor House.

Case One: Stevie

Stevie, age 13, was admitted to our residential program because his father had assaulted him in the schoolyard. His parents were divorced and in continual conflict. His family had reported more than 33 episodes of family violence to the police over the previous eight years. Stevie was one of four siblings ranging in age from eight to 15.

Prior to coming to our program, Stevie and his 11-year-old brother had been in several out-of-home placements. He presented with a large number of behavior problems, including expulsions from school, charges for car theft and burglaries, and vandalism in the community, especially the school.

Step One: All Stakeholders Together

As we developed the IST/RBA model, our staff members were deeply engaged. Referrals came into Windsor House for struggling young persons, and the preparation began in earnest. All stakeholders were identified early on, and the team was ready for new members to emerge over time. Each member agreed to use the same terminology. Not one stakeholder could be left out of the plans for the young person, especially in the beginning. This was, of course, a challenge, and there was not a "Doodle poll" to make coming together easier; it was hard work to make this happen. Attending were family members (including extended family), social workers, school counselors and teachers, a court liaison appointee, peers, mentors, and, of course, the identified young person. This step, that all stakeholders should be involved with the change agenda, created a collaborative plan of action. The therapist's use of Joining when working with families, from the outset, is even more important as the therapist brings stakeholders together. In Stevie's family, there had been "bad blood" with the agencies represented at the table; the mother had been placed as a young girl by social services and was still hurt and bitter. The father, who had been in and out of prison, had difficulty looking at the policeman who sat across from him.

Step Two: Stakeholders Determine the Objectives

The team started with the end (what they wanted to achieve) and worked backward in the practice of RBA. All stakeholders agreed on common outcomes and collaborated on the steps to achieve those outcomes. The real culture change was evident when work started and agreement was reached. Every component of the plan was weighed against whether it would lead to the goal of achieving agreed outcomes. IST posits that change occurs when the team functions as an organized system of care; their ready collaboration from the starting gate was confirming.

Step Three: IST/RBA Clinical Scorecard

The completion of the Scorecard by stakeholders was the fruit of their collaboration. The team used it for planning, tracking performance, and supervision. The data-rich tool enabled the treatment team to track this data transparently (Table 5.1).

It was a struggle getting the divorced, embattled parents to agree to be in the same room. Our partnership with the senior social worker, who had many years of experience with the family, facilitated the introductions. She was successful at convincing and, frankly, cajoling them to "come to the table." Using the New Zealand concept of "Cultural Safety," this Māori family was more comfortable working with our team because of the clinical team's inclusion of a kaumatua (Māori tribal elder). "Cultural Safety" is the family's sense of security in the clinical sessions. The kaumatua, a person highly regarded by the whanau (family), blessed the sessions and supported the family. "Cultural competence," valued in the United States, relates to the professional's knowledge of the client's culture.

Goal. The goal of "a well-functioning citizen" was the aspirational goal we established for Stevie and many of our youngsters. This might be considered by some too far a reach for these troubled and seemingly hopeless kids. But I cautioned the staff to be wary of self-fulfilling prophecies. You must firmly believe in the multi-faceted self. Change the context and Stevie will flourish.

Plans. Working backward from the goal, the team planned the steps for definitive change. The focus was the parents' embattled relationship, the engine that drove the instability. This poor hierarchy and triangulation maintained Stevie's lawlessness. Close collaboration was essential since the entire system needed to be congruent for success. Given the parents' explosive relationship, we were especially vigilant for any discord that might be created isomorphically among the stakeholders and may destabilize the system. Instituting the token economy, incentivizing Stevie to adhere to the rules, helped him focus on his daily behavior and he was rewarded weekly.

Measures. As I said, we adopted the CAFA. We considered it the gold standard for assessment and tracking outcomes. It focuses on function-ing: school, behavior toward others, mood/emotions, home, thinking problems, self-harm, substance use, and community. These domains, each a subscale, are behaviorally descriptive and anchored. The Team scored these subscales and tracked them against targets on the Clinical

Table 5.1 Clinical Scorecard for Stevie

Goal	Plans	Measures	Targets	HM
To be a well-functioning citizen	Family therapy	CAFAS scores	10% improvement over two months	Father
	Close collaboration between bio-parents, teachers, residential parents	School performance	Reading and math improve—one level in two months	
	Token economy activated with weekly payoffs	Token economy points	Points improved: 20% over two months	
	Discharge	Scores on the Triangulation or Single Parent's Scales	Triangulation Scale score decreased by 30% in three months	

Scorecard. Very importantly, this instrument gave the clinicians close feedback toward the effectiveness of our clinical program.

Stevie's excessive suspensions from school, resulting in falling behind, required great effort to bring him up to age-appropriate educational levels.

The token economy system is a time-honored behavioral therapy tool that rewards good behavior. It helps the youngsters focus on their immediate comportment. These points were accrued over short periods of time and weekly rewards were given by caregivers. It provides an opportunity to incentivize and shape good behavior.

The Triangulation and Single Parent's Scales addressed interactional patterns that are risk factors post-discharge. The Triangulation Scale measured the degree to which the young person was "caught" between two disagreeing primary caregivers and gauged the severity of the pattern. The Single Parent's Scale measured the social supports for the single parent and prompted the therapist to address the HM within the system.

Targets. The team set the best estimates of measures over time. These nodal points were important to assess progress, especially for a long-term residential program such as ours. A team can become easily lulled by the day-to-day routine.

Homeostatic maintainer. Certain members of a family system are more active in maintaining the status quo. In Stevie's family, when the therapist intervened to help the couple compromise, the father would not cooperate. We deemed him the homeostatic maintainer.

Turning the Curve: Tracking Performance over Time

The CAFAS score for three school terms (see Figure 5.1) indicated that Stevie was not improving; scores trended in the wrong direction. We viewed this therapeutic impasse as an indicator that we needed to redouble our efforts. There were two steps that the team considered: adding more intensity into the family therapy with the use of Unbalancing, or broadening the system. The clinical team met with the family, teachers, and partners, and recruited the grandmother who had been considered peripheral. We increased the intensity of our message and instituted more family therapy sessions.

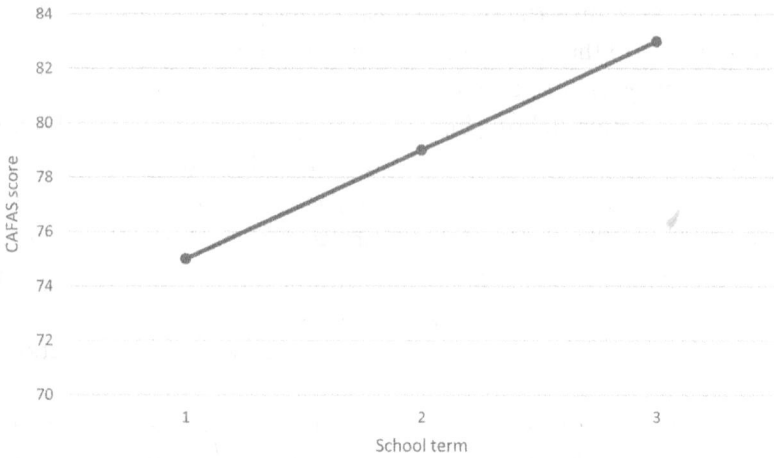

Figure 5.1 Graph of Stevie's CAFAS scores across three school terms (lower scores indicate better functioning).

The Triangulation Scale, during this three school term period (see Figure 5.2), indicated that triangulation was exacerbated. Again, this supported the need for redoubled efforts of treatment.

The Triangulation Scale scores and the CAFAS scores for the fourth and fifth school terms (see Figures 5.3 and 5.4) show marked improvement.

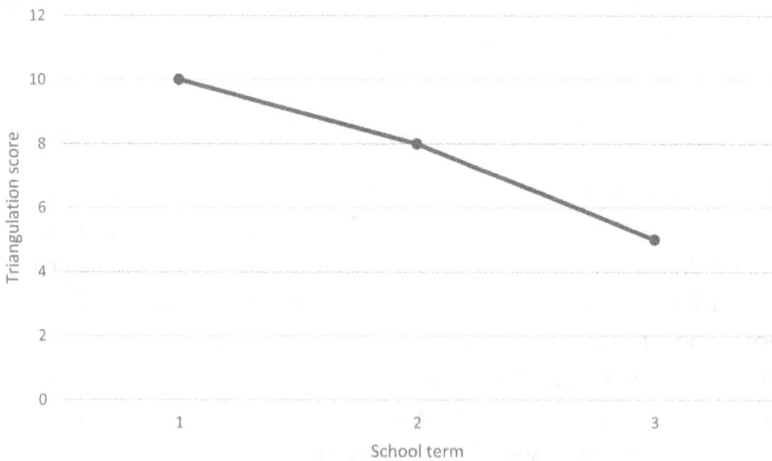

Figure 5.2 Graph of the triangulation scores between Stevie's parents across three school terms (higher scores indicate better functioning).

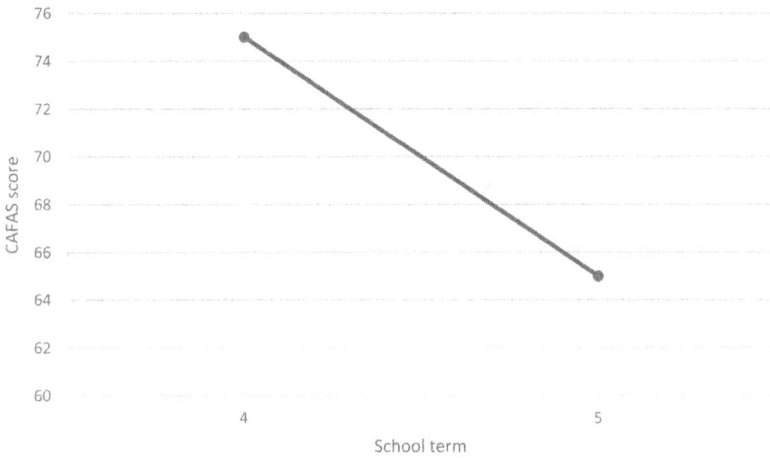

Figure 5.3 Graph of Stevie's CAFAS scores in the fourth and fifth school terms (lower scores indicate better functioning).

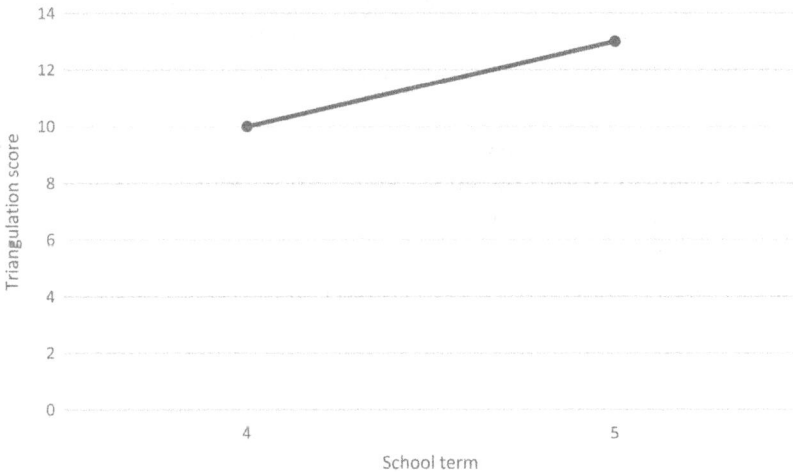

Figure 5.4 Graph of the triangulation scores between Stevie's parents in the fourth and fifth school terms (higher scores on the Triangulation Scale represent decreased triangulation).

Discharge

With the demonstrated improvement in the Triangulation Scale and the CAFAS scores, the clinical team determined that Stevie and his family were getting ready for discharge. When the slope of the triangulation scale shifted down, he was ready. That said, with economically disadvantaged families living in multi-problem communities, there were likely challenges ahead. A three-month follow-up was conducted; Stevie was well-functioning in the family and the community with occasional minor setbacks.

Composite Scores (Turning the Curves)

As clinicians and managers, we addressed the RBA question: Is anybody better off? We systematically collected data, tracked our progress, and documented it by using the Turning the Curve tool. Graphically displayed data relating to particular measures answered our important questions. We also used the Turning the Curve Tool to document the overall progress of the program with Composite Scores of the residents.

These scores for the CAFAS and Triangulation Scale scores (see Figures 5.5 and 5.6) improved over the five school terms (numbered 1–5 on the chart) for all the young people in our program. This was good news; this newly designed integrated IST/RBA model appeared to be effective.

The benefits of this amalgamated model include collaborative goal setting, individualized measures, the Clinical Scorecard, and most importantly, the addition of the identification of the homeostatic maintainer. Together, these components help to ensure that all members of the team are clear about the treatment and that interventions are targeted to achieving the desired outcomes.

Case Two: Billy

Billy, a 14-year-old male, who had become increasingly out of control starting at age ten, entered our program. His family was unable to control his behavior, and the police wanted him out of their small town.

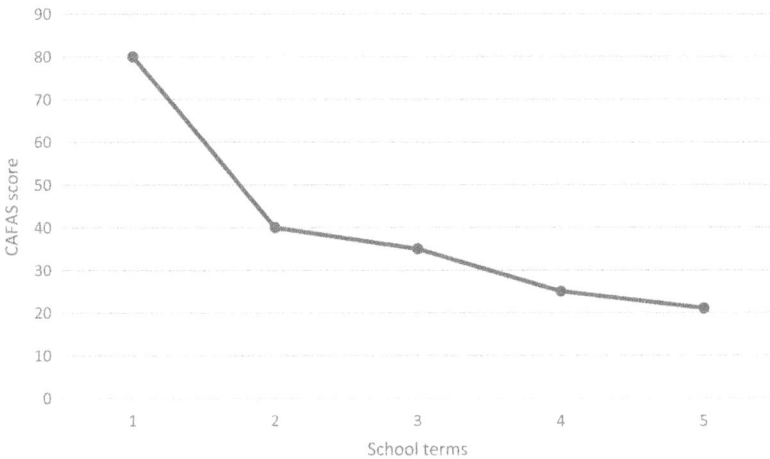

Figure 5.5 Average CAFAS for clients across five school terms (lower scores represent better functioning).

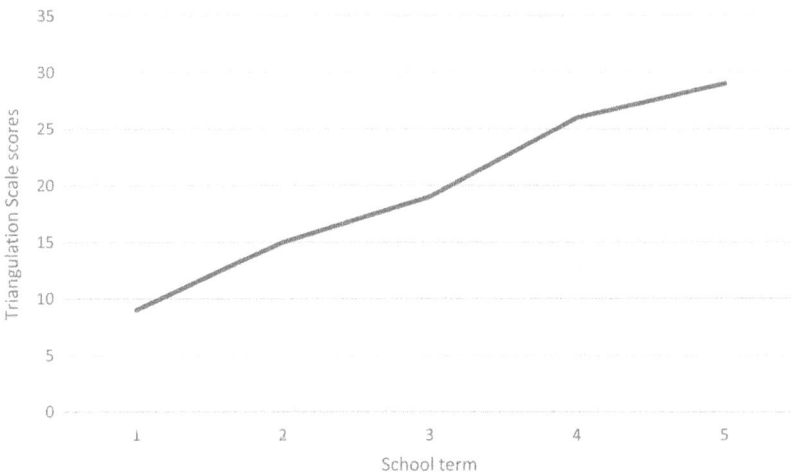

Figure 5.6 Average Triangulation Scale scores for clients across five school terms (higher scores predict better functioning).

Billy was involved in burglaries and was a heavy drug and alcohol abuser. Prior to treatment, Billy lived with his parents. When he attended school, he was repeatedly sent home early for "bad behavior." In addition, after searching his bedroom, his Mum, Shelley, and Dad, Tim, discovered stolen property from car thefts. Challenged during the first family therapy session, Billy, in response, assaulted a staff member. Our offices were on lockdown for most of the day while the police attended to the incident.

Billy's family rallied together and was consistent in attending the family therapy sessions. The therapist reported that his family worked hard to implement changes in the "system" and followed through with recommendations. The father changed his job from timber harvesting—climbing giant trees deep in the forest; he left home at 4.00 am and returned at 8.00 pm exhausted. To be more available to the family, he shifted his work to residential gardening. As the family system began working together and implementing changes, Billy's behavior gradually improved. He started to set goals for himself, and it wasn't long before it dawned on him that changing his behavior led to good things in his life.

Billy began to spend most of his free time on weekends and holidays with his family—which was incident-free. He no longer stole other people's property, and he changed his peer group to less toxic kids. He also started taking pride in his appearance. He started looking forward to the future, a manifestation of his improved self-esteem.

The CAFAS score and the Triangulation Scale indicated that Billy was ready to be discharged. His CAFAS went from 150 to 0; he was functioning well in all domains. Equally important, his Triangulation Scale (mother and father) similarly went in a positive direction (approximately from 15 to 30). By the time Billy was discharged, the mother was quoting from a family therapy text that the therapist had loaned her.

Follow-up at Three Months

The parents reported that Billy appeared to be thriving. He was planning to enroll in a military academy at the start of the next year and hoped this would lead to a career serving his country. The parents enjoyed their new work schedules and their "new son" (Figures 5.7 and 5.8).

Follow-up at 12 Months

This family attended in person for a follow-up session; they reported that things continued to improve. Billy was doing well at military school, and he was now involved with multiple community groups and sports teams. He was even going to the gym regularly. The most positive part was that

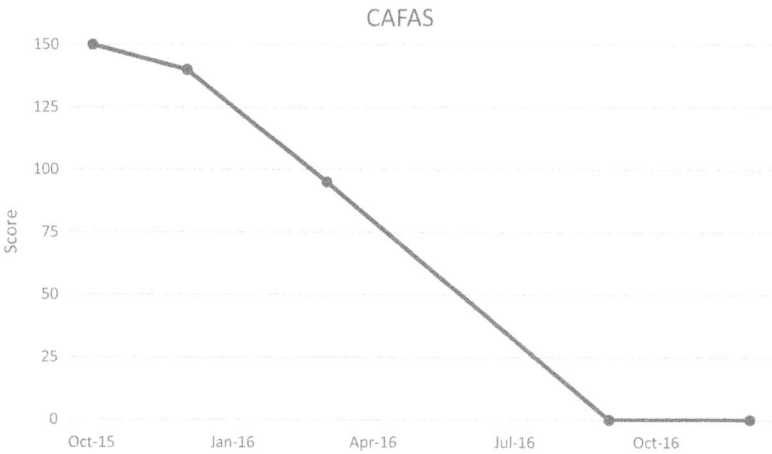

Figure 5.7 Billy's CAFAS scores from October 2015 to October 2016.

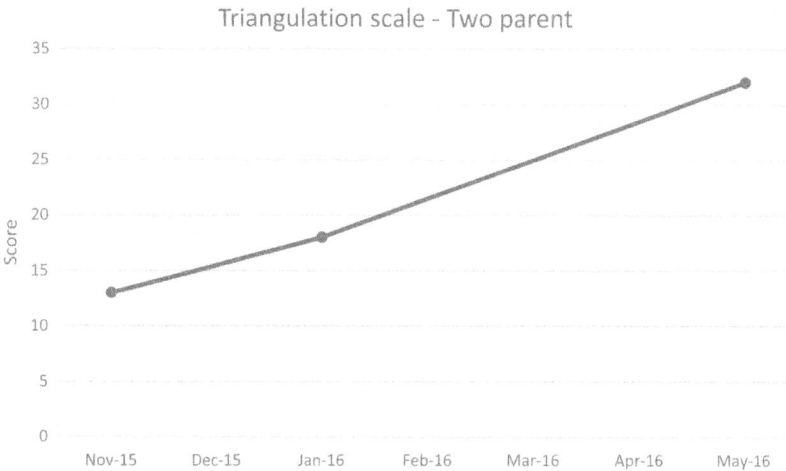

Figure 5.8 Billy's Triangulation Scale scores from November 2015 to May 2016.

Billy's positive changes appeared to be rubbing off on his siblings, who were also participating in a lot of the activities.

Case Three: Amber

A colleague of mine, who was instituting changes in her primary care clinic, asked if she could try the Clinical Scorecard Tool to manage one of her diabetic patients.

Amber, a 23-year-old Pacific Islander, sought help from her family practitioner because of obesity and type 2 diabetes mellitus. Amber was enrolled in the nurse-led diabetic clinic but her nurse was not comfortable or skilled in working with the larger family. Amber lived at home with her parents and five younger siblings, and her own three children, ages four, two, and one; a crowded house with few boundaries. All were enrolled in this same general practice clinic. She left school at age 15, pregnant, with little direction, and no plans for further education or training.

In the home, as the oldest, she was responsible for much of the care of her younger siblings as well as her own three children. She presented as despondent and defeated, and indicated that she felt trapped by her childcare responsibilities. "I have no life," she said. "I'm hopeless. I am trapped at home with my own children and siblings. My only relief is in the fridge—I can't bother about diabetic control." Amber's parents disagreed on whether Amber should attempt to get additional schooling/ training; one parent was concerned about the overall loss of child care. The triangulation was evident (Table 5.2 and Figure 5.9).

The immediate advantage of using the IST Clinical Scorecard in this setting was that the family stress leading to this young woman's weight gain and subsequent diabetes exacerbation was addressed. A clinical psychologist provided the family therapy in the clinic. The initial goal was for Amber to be well-functioning in all essential psychosocial domains, not just the medical ones. Furthermore, using the Scorecard, all stakeholders coordinated efforts around the agreed-upon goals and markers to access progress and performance. The use of the targets increased the sense of urgency for the team to push for change as well as to track progress. The medical team could track short- and long-term outcomes as care progressed. These measurable intermediary goals were essential in the treatment of chronic problems such as obesity and diabetes. All clinical eyes were focused on the Scorecard; it created a common language, transparency, and shared responsibility.

The general practitioner and the clinical team valued the Scorecard and, for many, it was the first time they had witnessed the importance of expanding the patient's context in clinical care. To implement this Tool as a standard would, unfortunately, require a change in the funding pathway and this posed challenges to this clinic.

Table 5.2 Clinical Scorecard for Amber

Objectives	Plans	Measures	Targets	HM
To be functioning well (biopsychosocially)	Improve diabetes control	HbA1c (mmol) monthly	20% reduction in HgbA1C over three months	Mother
	Fitness "Big Girls" Program; weight loss	Attendance to program (2 × wk); weight (kg)	Weight loss of 6 kg in three months	
	Family therapy—stress reduction	Score on Triangulation Scale	20% improvement in triangulation in three months	
	Vocational / educational counseling	Plan developed		

Amber HbA1c levels

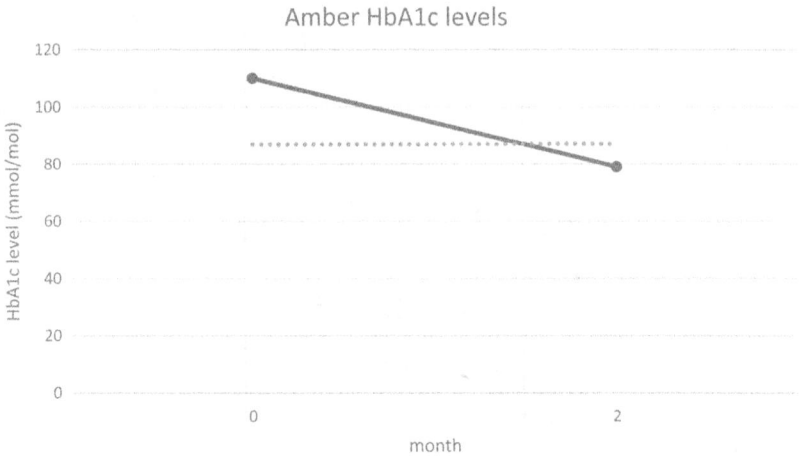

Figure 5.9 Amber's blood glucose (HbA1c) levels per month in treatment, measured in mmol/mol. The red line indicates her three-month target (87).

This case has been included to demonstrate the usefulness of these ideas with different patient populations, not just troubled adolescents.

Case Four: JD

I include this case to demonstrate some of the usefulness of Turning the Curve in yet a different clinical context.

I was consulted by a psychiatric Fellow on the case of JD, a 15-year-old boy with hyperemesis—extreme, excessive, and persistent vomiting that led to dehydration, electrolyte imbalances, and possible malnutrition. This very unusual symptom, usually associated with weight loss, is generally seen in pregnant women. The youngster had had many emergency department visits and subsequent hospitalizations in the past year. The Fellow said, "I believe he's currently hospitalized again for the 14th time."

I asked about the divorced parents. According to the Fellow, "The parents can't stand to be in the same room with each other, will not sit on the same couch together, nor will they even look at each other." There was pressure from the medical consultants to do more tests, even though the boy had undergone extensive medical evaluation. Prior to this meeting, I charted his ER visits to establish a Curve over time (see Figure 5.10).

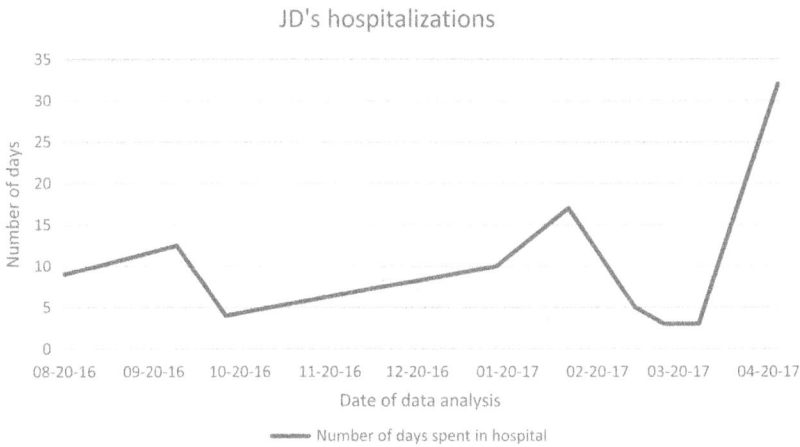

Figure 5.10 JD's hospitalizations over nine months.

There was a curious two weeks around March 20, 2017, when the hospitalizations approached zero. I inquired, "What was different during these weeks?" I was told that family therapy was conducted during that period. With this evidence and the power of a simple graph, the family and the medical team agreed to continue therapy before launching more investigations. The youngster improved with this approach.

Conclusion

In our residential program, we used the IST/RBA framework to considerable advantage for our consumers, staff, and other stakeholders. Straightforward, transparent, and practical, it facilitated the creation of a data-driven service that enhanced the organization of the young person's and family's entire system around outcomes—from the onset of treatment.

In our own search of the literature, we found scant data to address the crucial question of when to discharge. We found that our key parameters accurately helped to address this question: if the scores on the CAFAS were low, and the family markers of the Triangulation or Single Parent's scores were high, then the team was more confident in discharging the adolescent from the program.

IST/RBA's focus on grounded data and the use of Turning the Curve and the Clinical Scorecard enabled our clinicians and teams to determine the effectiveness of their clinical model.

RBA and IST have much in common as complementary frameworks. Both are change initiatives seeking to establish clear goals at the onset. These frameworks need each other for enduring systems change. Struggling on the front line with the broader system can be hard on your elbows. The corollary, piling on services, while not addressing the war at the center of the family, will not lead to change.

6

RBA/IST FOR EATING DISORDERS

The Johnny Appleseed of objectives and key results (OKRs) has been bestowed to John Doerr, a protégé of Andy Grove. In the early days of the computer revolution, Grove, a Hungarian immigrant who had fled Hitler, started at Intel, a small company destined to become a world leader in computer chip manufacturing. Grove later became CEO, and he managed the company using the principles of OKRs. His method of management and leadership helped him to establish Intel as the world's largest chip manufacturer at the time. In the process, he became the father of management science.

John Doerr started at Intel as an intern. His experience of working with Grove embedded a deep respect and understanding of the effectiveness of his OKR management; using these ideas, he rose to a senior management position. After some years, he left and became a venture capitalist, teaching OKRs to emerging companies.

Along the way, he wrote the book *Measure What Matters* (2018), borrowing the ideas from Grove's management style. He stated in his book

DOI: 10.4324/9781003161257-7

that the team should identify what matters (their objectives) and then find ways of measuring progress toward those objectives through specific measurable key results. They should be written down (transparent) and shared with everyone to instill collaboration. Doerr admitted, "They were not easy to do." He did say that when they are implemented faithfully, and get adopted, the system always works; he had never seen it fail. He further suggested that his principles of management and measuring could be applied to any company, agency, or organization.

When they were still working in their dorm room, Doerr taught the founders of Google, Larry Page and Sergey Brin, the OKR management philosophy for their fledgling company. They adopted the ideas immediately. Doerr was so impressed with how they embraced the ideas that he purchased 11% of the company (Doerr, 2018).

The OKR, a simple idea, has helped many for-profit companies reach a net worth in the billions; RBA, also with a simple idea, has saved governmental agencies across the world probably billions of dollars. Profits for some; savings for others. The simplicity of their messages and the focus on measuring what matters were considered innovative or, in popular speak, disruptive.

The ideas in this book may well be within this "simple message" framework. The clinical problem in front of a clinician requires measurable scales that matter; they are easily developed when using grounded observations and can be tracked over time. These scales are often on a PRN (as needed) basis, and you should not have to twist the situation to meet validation demands of academia that may be removed from what is going on at the front line. If you are working within an organization, then collaboration and transparency should be applied to establish accountability.

Eating disorders (ED) are not for the faint of heart; they are dangerous and expensive. The Strategic Training Initiative for the Prevention of Eating Disorders engaged Deloitte Access Economics to estimate the social and economic impact of EDs in the United States in 2018–2019. The total financial costs associated with ED were estimated to be $64.7 billion. The health system costs were $4.6 billion, with Americans out of pocket by $363.5 million. EDs were associated with 1.3 million disability-adjusted life years (DALYs) in 2018–2019, which represents a value of $326.5 billion (Deloitte Access Economics, 2020).

In 2015, Beat, the UK's eating disorder charity, commissioned Price Waterhouse Cooper (PwC) to estimate the costs of the social, health, and economic impacts on eating disorders. They estimated the cost to society was circa £15 billion per annum. Based on prevalence estimates, and assuming a ratio of one carer to one sufferer, an annual direct financial burden of between £2.6 billion to £3.2 billion was determined. Total treatment costs to the NHS was £3.9 to £4.6 billion; private costs were £0.9 to £1.1 billion; lost income to the economy was between £6.8 and £8 billion. The costs sit alongside the broad personal impacts: over 90% of the surveyed respondents reported a very significant or significant impact on their wellbeing and quality of life (PwC, 2015).

For more than half of the sufferers, the recurring cycle of treatment, recovery, and relapse (requiring repeat treatment) lasts for more than six years. The full size of these issues and confirming the prevalence rates of EDs need further exploration (PwC, 2015).

The Butterfly Foundation, an Australian organization that provides support for Australians who suffer from eating disorders, in 2014, released findings from their report *Investing in Need: Cost-Effective Interventions for Eating Disorders*. The report determined that it can cost more than $100,000 to appropriately treat a person with anorexia; if someone has anorexia for a decade (which happens often, since EDs are long-lasting and debilitating conditions), the costs of their foregone productivity and other financial costs would be larger. The total cost, if "treatment as usual" occurs, for those who developed an eating disorder in 2014 was equivalent to $103.2 billion, but the total cost, if "optimal treatment" occurs, was equivalent to $49.9 billion (net present value over ten years) (Hamilton, 2016).

Anorexia Nervosa

People with anorexia nervosa (AN) are 18 times more likely to die by suicide, and those with bulimia nervosa (BN) are seven times more likely to die by suicide, relative to gender and age-matched comparison groups (Smith et al., 2018). Anorexia nervosa is the most fatal disease per capita of the mental health diseases (Insel, 2012).

Here's a look at what's commonly involved in treating people with anorexia. Hospitalization, if life is at risk, and other programs (some residential), along with medical care (monitoring of condition), restoring a healthy weight, and psychotherapy that may include FBT and CBT. There are no medications approved to treat anorexia; none have been found to work very well (NHS, n.d.).

Having treated eating disorders for many decades, I am incredulous that the literature continues to report such staggering costs and horrific dangers. This does not have to be. The simple solution I described in my book, Enduring Change in Eating Disorders: Interventions with Long-Term Results (Fishman, 2004), is to assess the system and treat quickly the underlying structural components of the family system that are maintaining the symptoms. It is effective and inexpensive. In the tradition of science, following the success of previous generations, I chose my model of treating EDs based on the Psychosomatic Family Model of Salvador Minuchin as discussed earlier. I focus on Triangulation and Conflict Avoidance from among the tenets of the model since they are the most accessible to the therapist and the most potent. Others like rigidity and overprotectiveness do not have the same immediate accessibility. Focusing on these interactional patterns, powerful levers, facilitates the restructuring the young person's context.

Self-starvation, purging, and/or compulsive overeating are the symptoms of these diseases. They broadcast the underlying contextual isomorphic patterns that lead to the expression of these symptoms. Treating those patterns successfully decreases symptomatology.

In AN, it is their non-congruent context, usually their triangulating parents, that activates and maintains the symptom. Similarly, with BN and compulsive overeating (COE), the underlying pattern is conflict avoidance that maintains symptoms. Correct the pattern, and the dangerous behaviors mitigate. These are simple, observable markers that are readily measured by the clinician and, especially, the sufferer. "Measure what matters," from Mark Friedman and John Doerr, filters down from government agencies and mega-corporations to front-line mental health care and efficiently transforms family suffering.

Case One: Maria

Maria, 16 years old, with flaming red hair and a shrunken body, stared at me. She had been suffering from anorexia for six months. During that time, she had lost 25 pounds and ceased to menstruate while exercising compulsively. She would alternate between aggressive outbursts and paralyzed dysphoria. During one of her inpatient admissions, the nurse found her on the floor of a closet with a plastic bag over her head. She spent six months in the public health system; she was fed via nasogastric intubation with each of three hospitalizations. Upon discharge, back at home, the self-starvation would resume, leading to re-hospitalization.

She was referred to me by her grandmother, who had heard about my anorexia treatment from a neighbor. Maria's family had lost faith in the public hospital system. I remember the beginning of Maria's treatment; her petrified parents sat on either side of their daughter, fearing they were losing her.

Maria's parents had been divorced for 11 years. They had a tense relationship; the father was more interested in being Maria's friend than her parent, leading him to actively undermine the mother's parenting. The father functioned as the homeostatic maintainer. The mother would cajole her daughter to eat, the father would not cooperate. Prior to being referred to me, when Maria was in the hospital, the staff, not understanding the family systems model, saw the father as such an encumbrance for the remediation of Maria's anorexia that they sought to have a legal injunction forbidding him to enter the hospital.

I met with Maria and her parents to describe my approach, uniting the parents for the treatment ahead; this was uneventful. A few hours later, however, her mother called me and said Maria was out of control. Running out of the house into the street, agitated, crying uncontrollably. Because of her dangerously erratic behavior, I suggested the parents call the police, which they did. I heard no more from them that night. Calling me that morning, I was told that Maria had calmed down when the police visited. Our work began the next day. Family therapy immediately stabilized the system. The sessions focused on the parents working together, and from that point on, Maria ceased losing weight. The therapy continued—the complicated process of getting the father to effectively support the mother, who was slowly receptive to his help, was the task of the next few months. The father, in an alliance with his own mother, was recalcitrant. I worked closely with him, Joining, then challenging him to "get with the program" and support his ex-wife. It was a slow process.

Maria was weighed every three days. The father would come over to the mother's house and together they would engage in overseeing her eating.

If Maria had achieved her desired weight gain, she could attend school, and if not, she was assigned bed rest under the supervision of her parents, or her grandmother, should the parents be unavailable. Therapeutically, we attempted to find every possible situation in which the parents could demonstrate to the girl their willingness to function as a unit.

The Triangulation Scale, initially, reflected this 11-year family dysfunction. When the father refused to cooperate with the protocol, an exacerbation of the anorexia emerged; when the parents worked together, the food refusal abated. Maria's weight acted as a proxy for the degree of parental triangulation.

At the beginning of the treatment of eating disorders, I partner with the family and the young person to track the weight gain closely. This weight gain imperative serves as a lever for the parents to change, as well as monitoring the stability of the patient's medical condition. The Tool, *Weight Gain Personal Progress Guide*, is found on my website and is easily accessible for patients. It can also be located in the Appendix of this book.

This approach conforms to the IST/RBA Model: measuring weight over time and monitoring family structural changes (observable grounded interactions) in the areas of de-triangulation. Weight gain is a metric for tracking the parents' progress in working as a unit and the amelioration of the starvation (Figure 6.1).

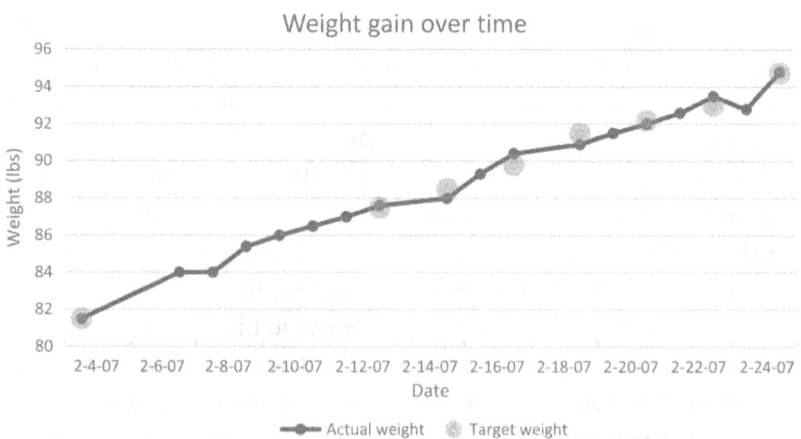

Figure 6.1 Maria's Turning the Curve.

Two-Year Follow-up

Maria's parents united; triangulation was abated. She gained 17.6 pounds, which was her agreed-upon target weight.

Maria's Parents' Narrative at the Last Session of Treatment (Transcribed)

Father: Yeah, it's the hardest thing I have ever had to experience in my life and the most emotional that I have ever been. It has also taught me a lot about myself because I have been too soft, you know, and not realizing in the beginning that it's a different person and you could lose your child, you know? The Maria that we knew as a happy, lovely, bubbly child, friendly and social, disappeared; she would bang her head against the wall, put a plastic bag over her head to try to kill herself, her mantra was, "I just want to die, I just want to die," you know? She would try to jump out of moving cars, try to jump off a deck. You said that she would come right in time, once the weight was on, but you kind of only understand it intellectually. Once you see that light come on, once the weight is back on, it's like my child is back and she's in the kitchen singing, asking how was your day and giving us a hug, you know? It's like; you don't believe that you are actually going to get your child back because you are living in such a negative vibration for such a long time, and then all of a sudden it's there, you know, all of a sudden there's light at the end of the tunnel, you know, you walk around with a broken heart all the time.

Mother: The power is in us two working together, that's the recovery, that's what's important. And what a struggle it was!

I live in a small town. At various points, I bump into Maria or one of her family members. Anorexia, according to her parents, ceased completely after treatment. She is pursuing a career in design at a university in another part of New Zealand.

Ironically, anorexia is a disease of the well-fed, of the middle and upper classes. These families do not have a complicated array of social

service agencies involved in their lives unlike the economically disenfranchised. Initially, a destabilizing component that made this particular
case more complicated was Maria's paternal grandmother, despite having
referred the family. Over time, her support of the therapy became an
important asset. Additionally, the primary care physician was an invaluable partner in the treatment; he monitored Maria's physical health and
provided timely collaboration.

Note: There is a bed-rest protocol in the Appendix.

Bulimia Nervosa (BN) and Compulsive Over Eating (COE)

In the treatment of BN and COE, the targeted interactional pattern of
conflict avoidance is measured and tracked. My theory of change posits
that when conflict is avoided, the symptom emerges. The corollary is
also true: if the sufferer successfully addresses the conflict, the purging
and compulsive over eating diminish.

The patients tend to present as young adults and sometimes older. The
majority of these patients are female, with men comprising at most 25%
(Weltzin et al., 2005). They have larger, more complicated social systems
and families that at times are continents away. I treated one woman who
was in her mid-70s; surprisingly, in spite of the 50-year marriage, she
stopped purging once she began confronting her husband.

In terms of the concept of conflict avoidance, I still remember
a comment made to me many years ago by Virginia Satir, a social
worker who is considered among the early pioneers of family therapy.
A visionary, Virginia introduced conjoint couples' therapy to psychotherapy. Referring to psychosomatic symptoms, she said, "The
body says what the mouth won't" (personal communication, 1980).
Indeed, the compulsion to purge is inversely correlated to what's not
being said.

The BN and COE Worksheet measures purging incidents, overeating,
and conflict avoidance episodes; they are tracked weekly. In using this
Tool, each time an individual experiences a stressful interaction and feels
like purging/bingeing, she notes what conflict or area of procrastination she is experiencing. Procrastination, putting off what the person

has intended to do, becomes an intra-personal conflict, in fact conflict avoidance. The Worksheet gives the client the correlation between conflict avoidance and their symptoms. Each week the patient notes their results and determines their total Conflict Score Response. The theory of change with both of these behaviors is the patient confronting conflictual relationships.

It is important to emphasize that the sufferer's insight regarding the association between conflict or procrastination and their symptom is not enough. This is not an insight therapy. It is a therapy focused on changing an interactional pattern that is maintained by the meta-rule of rules in their psychosomatic families and broader contexts. The patient must act, come face to face with the conflict, and work to resolve their bubbling discomfort.

The Bulimia Nervosa and Compulsive Overeating Worksheet is found in the Appendix. At the onset of treatment, this tool is downloaded from the Tools for Change section of my website.

Case Two: Janice

Janice, 29 years old, was a sailor. The weekend before our session, she had taken a group of friends out sailing. Highly experienced, she was the captain, but her guests ignored new leadership. Furious, rather than trying to corral them by asserting herself, Janice took refuge in the galley, purging repeatedly. In the course of our work together, she began addressing the conflictual relationships in her life, such as her overprotective family and her friendships. The data from the Worksheet helped her to see the pattern—conflict avoidance leading to purging.

Case Two: Hannah

Hannah, aged 30, severely bulimic, lived with her long-term partner. When the partner entertained his friends at home, he expected Hannah to tidy the kitchen and clean the house at the end of the evening, while he would go to bed. She was furious but said nothing to him. Instead, she purged. The Worksheet exercise over the weeks of her therapy provided the understanding that her relationship with her partner exacerbated her symptoms. She arrived the next week with her partner in tow and confronted him in the session. Through this initiative, they began to transform their relationship. Her purging episodes ceased.

Case Three: Belle

Belle, a 23-year-old woman, had manifested bulimia for six years. In her email requesting an appointment, she said she was desperate and hopeless, nothing had worked. She had seen "countless therapists," and nobody made a difference. I began with the usual question, "What needs to change?" and received the customary answer, "I need to change. Food is driving me crazy." As is my practice at the commencement of treatment, I suggested the problem with eating disorders is not food, but it's your relationships. Belle and I explored the people in her life. She had a tormented relationship with her family; she experienced both parents as intrusive and disparaging.

The next week when she came in, she told me that she hadn't purged, and she had held her ground with the various people in her life, especially her father. We discussed her history of romantic relationships. She said that she had had many experiences and had not been able to maintain a long-term relationship with a man. She said frequently there would be things in the relationship that bothered her, but she would always be afraid to bring them up. She would just "stew" and then bolt. She confided in me that she was a "sugar baby" with a "sugar daddy"; he supported her, in part, and they met irregularly to reduce suspicions from his wife.

In the process of our work, she learned that the way to have a truly intimate relationship was to honestly address those issues that she had so fastidiously avoided. She wanted to free herself of her ignominious position of being a "kept" woman. She began in earnest to develop a career, all the while paying close attention to her Worksheet. She became a successful real estate agent and no longer suffered in silence. In her note, announcing her new agency, she mentioned her romantic partner of two years. She reported that she is happy and enjoying success.

Compulsive Overeating

Conflict avoidance is the pattern that maintains the behavior of COE. In BN and COE, it is always the same struggle. The patient is firmly convinced that the problem is food; I'm strongly convinced otherwise. The problem is relationships and, moreover, with COE, my patients have reported boredom and severe isolation. Boredom has attributes of procrastination, and isolation can be the result of avoiding conflict.

Case: Karen

Karen, a 49-year-old woman, had struggled with obesity for years. When we began working, she was 100 pounds overweight. An intelligent woman, Karen helped her husband manage their dairy farm. Few friends and rarely socializing kept her close to the refrigerator. She reported, "I have tried everything to lose weight."

Karen recognized that her interpersonal conflicts led to her compulsive overeating. Using the Worksheet, Karen noted that every time her eating became out of control, there was an association to a stressful interaction. In this case, it was usually within her family. For example, when her daughter-in-law would drop in, requesting, "Can you take care of my kids for an hour?" and then returned five hours later, Karen stayed silent and tight-lipped. As soon as the younger woman left, Karen would lose control of her eating.

With her husband, distant and "lazy," Karen's responsibilities on the farm were growing out of control. Her body spoke for her; she would binge.

The Worksheet confirmed very quickly to Karen that the conflicted relationships were making her fat. Developmentally, a big birthday, her 50th, was looming. She said she was terrified. She talked of "more than half-my-life is over." "Her knees would not likely get her into her sixties." The results of the Worksheet were proof and she began to hold her ground. She negotiated with her husband about farm-related responsibilities. She mandated new terms of reference with her daughter-in-law. According to Karen herself, she was "liberated" and "frisky"; charging ahead and facing conflict.

Follow-up Letter from Karen (Transcribed)

I just wanted to touch base and let you know how I am getting on. I am doing fantastic! I'm feeling pretty pleased with myself! I am using all the info you and I talked about regarding using my voice and being honest about voicing feelings, emotions, and situations instead of eating them! I continue losing weight. This has been a great help. I feel great! My food management is going along well, and I cannot remember the last time I ate so healthily! I have not binged, fasted, or over-eaten for the past year. I feel I now have the knowledge to deal with situations that arise in my life in a proactive manner rather than to suppress how I feel by stuffing my feelings down with food.

When I first began our therapy, I could not have imagined that I would ever be able to describe myself as anything but broken. But, now, a year and a half later, I feel that all of the words above describe how I feel about myself now.

I am quietly and confidently taking care of myself. My husband and I are happier, socializing more, and making new friends. I've lost 65 lbs. I am happy. It's not all smooth sailing, some weeks are better than others, but that's life and I now cope with the ups and downs in much more constructive ways.

Conclusion

I author my own tracking instruments by respecting the tradition of valuing the simplicity in the management systems of OKRs and RBA. The repeated patterns of how people interact and what happens in front of you allows easy codification. Your eyes tell you that the interactions you recorded are true and correct. The instruments are practical and helps clinicians predict family functioning and the next steps. These common-sense scales kick start the local clinical scientist to 'measure what matters.'

Last year, a 12-year-old girl was referred to me who had been severely anorectic for six months. She had been hospitalized in the local children's hospital where the treatment focused solely on her weight. As I reflected, it was basically a foie gras treatment—"stuffing the goose." The little girl reviled the intervention; it was so punitive. They were only interested in getting her to a target weight to discharge her from the hospital; the equivalent of "getting the goose to market."

Yes, in her $100,000-dollar medical treatment, they measured the weight parameter but ignored the other measurement that mattered. The simple solution that would free her and the family from the ravages of the tenacious anorexia was their moral imperative and they ignored it. They failed to measure the deep structures of her context.

The scientific tradition is based on building the advances of what came before from the work of one's predecessors. Even one of the most famous scientists in history has written, "If I have seen further, it is by standing on the shoulders of giants" (Newton, 1675).

7

THE COMMUNITY RESOURCE SPECIALIST

The sad truth! In highly troubled communities, such as those associated with Windsor House, even effective family therapy may not be enough to transform complex family systems. Isolation, poverty, racism, and marginalization will often interfere with a family's connectedness and functionality. Family therapy is necessary to properly address the myriad structural dysfunctions in the family; these issues are often found in the family microsystem. But, even then, it still may not be sufficient. The therapist will likely end up being an outsider, peeking in through the window shades of the family, without the leverage to transform the family's troubled broader system.

Andrea Banovcinova et al. reported in 2014 in the paper "The Impact of Poverty on the Family System Functioning" how life in poverty negatively impacts the functioning of the family system. With their methodology of using the McMaster Model of Family Functioning in their research, based on systems theory, the results showed that long-term economic stress led to less effective parenting. Parents often apply

DOI: 10.4324/9781003161257-8

coercive and punitive parenting styles more frequently, corporal punishments are frequently used, there is a higher risk of partner violence, and criminal behavior and addictive behaviors surface. The stress caused by constant economic pressure results in the instability of family relationships (Banovcinova et al., 2014).

Social isolation, described by Kim Samuel, is especially harmful when it is chronic, enduring over a long time (Synergos, n.d.). Feelings of shame and humiliation often accompany the isolated person (Narayan et al., 2000a; Narayan et al., 2000b). Deprivation of social connectedness is a core dimension of poverty, according to The Samuel Family Foundation (Sen, 2000, pp. 4-5). Synergos Institute, in partnership with Kim Samuel, and in collaboration with Oxford University's Poverty and Human Development Initiative, is working to overcome isolation and deepen social connectedness. Through her leadership as President of the Samuel Family Foundation, Samuel's work and thinking have emerged in a research paper. She has suggested that social connectedness provides people with a sense of belonging, facilitates access to supports and opportunities to achieve improvements that are desired and valued, and results in tangible assets (Synergos, n.d.).

As the team at Windsor House worked to achieve excellent outcomes with their young persons, their acknowledgment of their limitations in dealing with the poverty-related problems of the families precipitated desperation. Almost in unison, they chanted, "We need a specialist for this job." They were increasingly aware that they were unskilled in this area of helping, despite the many years of working with the population.

My experience in the early 1990s with the New Jersey School-Based Youth Services Program (SBYSP), which functioned as a "one-stop social services unit" for schools in the state's most troubled communities, lingered in my mind during the early years of my directing services at Windsor House. Roberta Knowlton, MSW, with the vision of a hundred eagles and falcons, developed and directed this New Jersey program. At one point, Roberta asked me to consult with some of the families who were in danger of having their child placed by court order into a residential placement. It was a sizzle to work with Roberta; she was always thinking ahead and out of the box. She had become increasingly aware of the power of family therapy after attending some of my training sessions in the area. She told me, "Our school-based programs are excellent, yet something is lacking. We are not working with their families—these struggling kids need family therapy" (personal communication, 1992).

I replied, "Family therapy would be an important addition, but, with families that are so economically disadvantaged and so often isolated in their ravaged communities, I fear it will not be enough." Grasping for ideas, I suggested that we needed someone from the families' communities to advocate for them—for better access to services; someone to walk alongside these families for support; and someone to tackle the insecurities of housing and food. This super-charged person would also need mettle to attend all manner of court-related infractions and charges that the family members were dealing with. Finally, employment opportunities had to be exhausted or created. My friends and families had tired of my obsession with "jobs" as a cure for most of what ailed these families. "J O B" had become my mantra to anyone who might listen; I did notice that my listening audience was dwindling. With that in mind, we agreed to develop a new position, the "community resource specialist" (CRS). We determined that the CRS would not only hail from the community but share the same ethnicity; we believed that it would enhance the cultural safety of the family and improve the cultural competency of the team. There was no formal qualification or educational attainment that was required; we worried that credentials might impede the organic activity required for this role. Credentials for this individual seemed simple— common sense, gumption, tenacity, and probably righteous indignation.

The position was advertised, and a first CRS was quickly hired. On the first day, she was invited to complement the standard family therapy assessment process, exploring with the family their extenuating social difficulties. The family therapist was focused on the immediate relationships within the family; the broader contextual issues, such as housing, employment, medical challenges, and finances, were situated within the portfolio of the CRS. It was discovered, after probing the details of an out-of-control teenager, that he lacked supervision from his father who had recently suffered a stroke. The CRS intervened quickly; she resourced an outpatient rehabilitation program for this deflated father. This invaluable program increased the father's confidence and physical functioning, making him more available to his son with renewed authority.

New Jersey is a state that houses great wealth in some areas, and profound poverty in others. A number of New Jersey cities, such as Trenton, Camden, and Newark, are former industrial powerhouses. On a trip from New York through to Trenton, I recall seeing an ironic banner as the train crossed the Delaware River: "Trenton makes, and the world takes." When I visited Newark, it was clear that time had passed this city by, leaving collapsed factories and derelict neighborhoods, rampant with poverty and the expected sequelae. In the mid-1990s, the epidemic of HIV further compounded the community's problems. Some parents died leaving their children parentless; others felt the burden of parenting while extremely ill. For many of the youngsters, school was a refuge. The harsh realities of their lives, especially the fulminant poverty, were mitigated by the school-based program in many ways.

Adolescents entering high school for the first time were identified by Roberta as a vulnerable period for her youngsters. We discussed targeting family therapy interventions for this risky period. The families of the 1,000 new students were invited to the school in the evening to introduce the ideas and orient the families to this additional support program. Only two mothers courageously pushed the door open. In contrast, one private school in Philadelphia sent a note home to parents, "Please only attend your child's teacher conference once." We were eager beavers, developing solutions for families without consulting the very families that needed help; then, embarrassingly, we were critical of their lack of interest and engagement. The empowered CRS set us straight; this pathetic disconnect needed repair. She really understood the families and their challenges and it became obvious that they knew she would work for them. Their relationships grew strong and they traversed uncertainties and complexities together; she helped people move forward in their lives: jobs or better jobs (I still feel tremendous warmth when I think of her interest in this domain), improved housing, and a solid ability to interface with government agencies. Our CRS openly admitted that she had painstakingly learned to traverse these impediments herself. Her success was her ability to partner with a wide range of family configurations. She knew and respected the families in this community.

Reflecting on the many appointed CRSs, I recall a young man from the Newark community who had, in his previous life, dealt drugs. He was apprehended for drug use and feared a prison sentence that was to take 20 years of his life. "By some miracle," he told me, "I was released after two weeks. God gave me a second chance. I pledged to dedicate myself to helping troubled teens." He was tireless and worked day and night to improve the lives of distressed families.

After a few years, we conducted an evaluation of the effectiveness of the addition of a CRS in working with adolescents with behavioral problems in the New Jersey SBYSP (Fishman et al., 2001). The study sample of 131 New Jersey high school students and their families, from districts of socioeconomic need, some rural and some urban, were reviewed. Among those students who received both family therapy and the services of the CRS, 66% showed improvement at treatment termination, whereas those who received only family therapy showed 28% improvement. Ten weekly sessions, averaging one to two hours, had been designated for both groups; the group where the treatments were combined received 6.22 sessions on average; the family therapy group only received 3.75 sessions on average. CRS involvement appeared to have decreased the attrition rate by nearly 40%.

I pretended for a few weeks that I could continue my work with this program, despite my acceptance and commitment to the Annie E. Casey Foundation Fellowship that began in 1995. I was so reluctant to step away from this initiative; it had real energy and we were collecting evidence that we were making a difference. My conversations with Roberta were bittersweet as we discussed my future with her team. The solution, we discovered, was nestled in the souls of two committed family therapists residing in New Jersey: Hinda Winawer, MSW, and Norbert Wetzel, ThD. With enthusiasm, they agreed to step in and provide the family therapy component as I handed over the reins. They did a marvelous job. They expanded the program across the state into 20 schools—elementary, middle, and high schools throughout New Jersey. Their final report (Winawer & Wetzel, 2011) showed that 93% of the students involved in the program stayed in school and 83% graduated in eight of the programs at high school sites. They reported that the collaboration of the CRS with their family systems specialist (family therapist) made the program real and credible. Funding was withdrawn after 20 years as the government changed hands; a sad reality for many public servants. I remain indebted to Hinda and Norbert for their important work.

With my migration to New Zealand and now holding the position at Windsor House, the staff leaned into the discussions and sat ramrod straight as I introduced the CRS concept that had been so successful in the New Jersey School system; they were interested. They saw the proverbial light at the end of their dark tunnel. Getting the CEO and financial officer on board was perfectly in keeping with bringing everyone together to tackle problems. Approving this budgetary surprise required their "buy-in." I guided the discussions, "selling" at times the value-add of a CRS, someone who would work in tandem with the lead therapist and sit at the table with all of the stakeholders as Clinical Scorecards were developed and reviewed. There was quick interest and acceptance; the need was just so great. Approving a change to the budget, mid-year, does challenge organizations; however, no hand-wringing was initiated. Human resources was charged with developing the hiring specifications along with the clinical team. The advertisement stated clearly what the role required: a deep connection to the community, an ability to work with out-of-control young people, and skills in lifting families out of poverty by eliminating the socioeconomic factors that were holding them back. The ability to work independently and within the team was clearly stated.

It is with pleasure that I introduce Whaea (esteemed older woman) Rahera, our first CRS. She grew up and lives in a Māori community similar to those in which our Windsor families resided (Figure 7.1).

In her position of CRS, Rahera worked to transform the family's social context—the daunting, real-life issues that so harshly impacted their lives. Rahera was deeply valued by the clinical staff members, and they often said, "What would we do without Rahera and her life-altering resources?" She possessed access to the cultural and social capital within our families' community. She agreed to discuss some clinical anecdotes for this book, providing an authentic voice to her outcome-driven approach. Much like the 1990s Newark style of the CRS, she always worked toward an organized system of support around the client and their family. She asserted her independence and authority as an elder member of the Maori community with practiced success.

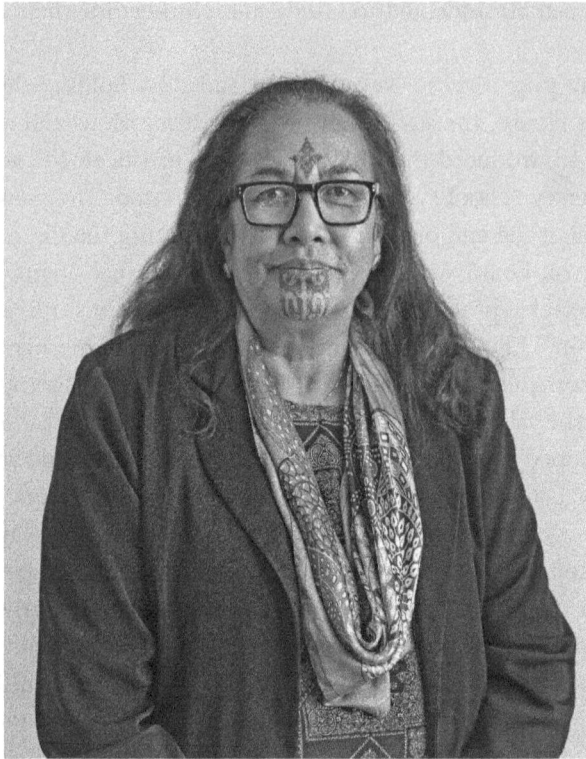

Figure 7.1 Rahera bears the *ta moko* (tattoo) that designates her Māori tribal identity.

In her voice, she leads us on the journey of two families and their complex worlds, helping to bring understanding and appreciation for the granular work of a CRS.

Case One: Justine

My first impression of Justine was her openness and warm smile. I recall her appearing distracted by my purple top and jacket throughout our first meeting. As we finished, she shared with me that purple was the color of "angels" in her faith, a color often worn by spiritual people.

She is a Māori mother of four, who has recently returned to New Zealand from Australia to take care of her children; they were previously living with her estranged husband. Her 12-year-old son had severe behavioral problems and was in our Windsor House residential program.

Justine and her children moved into the government-sponsored housing vacated by her husband. Two months into their stay, the government concluded that because her husband (the leaseholder) was no longer present in the household, the family had no grounds to occupy the home; they were to be evicted. Facing the prospect of homelessness, and unable to afford the rising rental prices in the city, Justine reached out to us. Unfortunately, our combined efforts to find suitable (safe, secure) accommodation for her family, at a price she could afford, were unsuccessful, and negotiations with government housing services proved fruitless.

Justine had very low self-esteem. She had a difficult time standing up for herself. In the past, she had allowed her husband to "take control" of everything and was now having a very hard time facing the major hurdles in front of her. I knew Justine for only a short time, however, I walked alongside her in every way that I could. My goal was to embolden her so she could take action and improve the circumstances for her family. Justine rose to the occasion. She courageously sought help from her local member of parliament. As a result, she was given a government house for her and her children.

Thankfully, we were able to link Justine to the following supports: City Women's Legal Advice (legal services); Food Bank Aotearoa (food and supplies); Citizen's Advice Bureau (advocacy); Supermarket Employment (current job). These support services helped Justine grow in confidence and she became more proactive when it came to any challenges that lay ahead. She was also better able to maintain family cohesion.

When I caught up with Justine two years later, she told me that she had filed for a divorce and was taking a course to help her obtain better job opportunities in the future. She shared with me that she was still working in a supermarket but was finally enjoying her life and able to "stand up for herself"; she saw this as a good indicator of a flourishing mauri (life force). She appeared to be embracing life, and her family was thriving.

Rahera's words bring this family to life; her modesty was her contribution and great power in bringing about change. As with most of our families, our goal was always to find ways to decrease the stress in the family members, especially the son, who was so out of control that he was mandated to our charge. The combined approach with a therapist leading the team and Rahera in tandem, expanding the universe of stakeholders and addressing the broader systemic challenges, ameliorated the problematic issues with Justine's son. We transformed the extracorporeal mind—in this case, the nuclear family plus the family's broader community.

Case Two: Bobbi

Bobbi is a Māori mother of two teenage boys and one adult daughter. Both of Bobbi's sons are in social service custody. Bobbi's younger son, Scott, is currently in our program. Bobbi lost her husband to cancer when the children were very young, however, it appeared she had not yet been able to move forward since his death. She still regularly imagined she was speaking with her deceased husband and shared with me her belief that her husband's death triggered the deterioration of her family.

Bobbi had been diagnosed with posttraumatic stress disorder (PTSD), which her family therapist believed was preventing her from seeking full-time employment. In lieu of a job, she was receiving unemployment benefits. During one session, Bobbi showed me a family photo taken just before her husband's death. Looking at it, I could not believe the changes since that time. The photo appeared to be of an average, middle-class, New Zealand family. Bobbi appeared happy, healthy, and emotionally stable, the complete opposite of how she currently appeared—frayed by hardship since her husband's passing.

The loss of the father was a turning point for the family system and it profoundly affected Bobbi. She clearly had not received the support she needed in the aftermath. One winter, in anger, she smashed three large living room windows in her house after receiving a letter indicating that she was behind on her rent. This left the family having to use trash bags to cover the holes and keep warmth in the home. I was able to support Bobbi in liaising with the landlord; he corrected an apparent error with the rent bill and agreed that he would replace the windows.

After her husband died, Bobbi became depressed. She found coping with activities of daily living very difficult. With her children in state care, she became nomadic, before ultimately being forced into public housing. She hated living there, so she isolated herself from other people. She also removed herself from family supports, feeling judged by family members.

In her community, Bobbi gained a reputation for being confrontational with service providers. During one serious incident, she made threats to social service workers, leading to her being barred from the social welfare office. As a result, most service providers refused to work with her, making it difficult for her to gain support and services for her and her children. Bobbi's antisocial behavior stemmed from her experiences with social service workers. She felt that they had only ever caused trouble for her family. She often voiced her concern that "people" were watching her, and she felt that her Facebook friends were spies who were sent to critique her Facebook posts. Her thought processes were often irrational and incoherent in this way. More importantly, she was often unable to accurately process information, which resulted in misunderstandings and conflicts.

My work with her progressed slowly. She didn't trust people. However, as I allowed her to "open up" at her own pace, trust developed between us. She perceived me as non-judgmental and an active listener. She eventually fully partook in our family resource services. During one of my visits, I found out that Bobbi's daily meals consisted solely of hot chocolate. Being estranged from medical and social services, she was not receiving medical care or food supplements.

She could not work because she was unwell. However, she had not yet been able to access the benefits available to her in New Zealand due to her untreated mental health. She remained devoted to her son's cat; she would not eat unless there was also food for the cat.

I asked her why she valued the cat so much, and she responded, "The cat is the only connection I have with my son."

I conveyed to the treatment team that Bobbi and her children needed support services in a variety of areas. We established a "strengths-based pathway toward improving her wellbeing," and that began with regular doctor's appointments with transport provided.

The enduring challenge was getting Bobbi to engage with a mental health service. She was intermittently enthusiastic, and I hoped that it would simply be a matter of my advocacy to ensure an assessment was completed. Bobbi remained ambivalent, however, and unfortunately, an incident resulted in her being legally mandated to engage [required to participate]. She threatened to harm a social worker after he showed up at her home unannounced, imploring her to sign documents allowing her son to live with his older sister and her family in Australia.

It is my belief that Rahera's success in forming a trusting relationship with Bobbi rested in their common Māori identity. She facilitated Bobbi's reconnection to her Māori community, her whakapapa (lineage). Her extended family provided a larger family for her children. She visited the marae (traditional meeting house) and her connections grew. The family of her deceased husband started to come into view.

Bobbi finally agreed for her son to move to Australia to live with his well-functioning grown sister and her family. Once this was accomplished, the focus was now centered squarely on his mother's wellbeing. Rahera worked to help build bridges between the sister and her mother, and this added assurance to the son that his mother was doing well. Rahera's practice in this case was closely aligned with the clinical team. This therapeutic system pulled together toward a specific goal—allowing Scott to move on with an important connection to his mother.

Rahera addressed Bobbi's mental health symptomatology by helping her secure a job. She broke it down into two simple steps: preparing a CV and completing applications. Her simplicity was her magic. In New Zealand, you are allowed and expected to bring a support person to your job interview, and Rahera served this important function. They had rehearsed interviewing and the parts each would play; Bobbi was well prepared. Rahera facilitated a vocational retreat with other family members who were seeking employment. She borrowed an idea from the Native American Indians (Māori feel a kinship to the indigenous people of the United States) and arranged a "sweat lodge" in her community—this novelty was a great success by all reports. Bobbi landed a job with a Māori service provider as a youth worker, and our team celebrated (Table 7.1).

An "Economic Opportunity Assessment and Intervention Tool" was developed by the team at Windsor House, along with Rahera, to help her with family assessments (see the Appendix). It served as a guide to help identify the family needs and potential interventions; each area was measured and the results were shared with the entire team. She was not limited by the Tool in her ability to seek resources. The "social determinants of health," established by the WHO in 2005 to support countries in addressing social factors that lead to health inequities, helped shape our tool. These determinants have gained global prominence over the years, and public policies now provide a clear lens for every citizen to be assessed for health equity. In New Zealand, in 2008, the Ministry of Health published *The Health Equity Assessment Tool: A User's Guide* (Signal et al., 2008). New Zealand believes that the social determinants of health are the circumstances and the environments in which people are born, grow up, live, learn, work, and age.

In naming our Tool, we inserted the area of focus (economics) and the area of action/interventions (opportunities) to remind the user to step quickly into a family and insert a change agenda. The Tool provided reminders and measurements for the work of the CRS. Rahera remarked about the importance of adding dates and updates. It gave her a perspective on the timeframes for developing relationships, collaborating with governmental agencies and courts, and embedding change. She was often disappointed by some of the data and the simple bare facts; she was well aware that the very poverty she was trying to address created immense barriers to her work with families: no transportation, no petrol, no current registration on the car, no access to Wi-Fi, mobile number changed without notification, lost or stolen mobiles, no computer, banned from libraries and governmental agencies, and bus passes expired. Just staying in touch with her families she found to be a daunting effort.

Table 7.1 Clinical Scorecard for Bobbi's son Scott

Objectives/goals	Plans	Measures	Targets	HM/barriers
Scott—well functioning	Help him move to live with the sister Facilitate mother's MH treatment—PTSD and paranoia Visits home and to sister Mother less isolated Mother getting a job	Mother in MH treatment Her psychiatric symptoms decreasing Improved relationship between mother and sister More social contacts for mom in her community Good working relationships for mom with doctors and social workers	Q/2 months access these plans	Mother—especially her mental illness

During the 1990s, while Hillary Clinton struggled to transform health care in America, Dr. Mary-Jane England, a child psychiatrist and director of the Washington Business Group on Health, a think-tank funded by Fortune 500 companies, developed a campaign. I remember this well since I was completing a Casey internship with this group during this period. The slogan Mary-Jane boldly advertised, "It's the system, stupid," emphasized that what was wrong with the health care system was the system itself (personal communication, 1995). She intended this slogan as a response to the belief that more money was the answer to health care reform. It lampooned Bill Clinton's slogan when he successfully challenged George H. Bush in the 1992 Presidential campaign, "It's the economy, stupid." It was not the individual practitioners or any specific group that was causing the health care system to go awry, it was the system itself, the systemic organization, the lack of organization!

In the United States, the National Technical Assistance Center for Children's Mental Health defined a System of Care in the following way: a spectrum of effective, community-based services and supports for children and youth with, or at risk for, mental health or other challenges and their families; that is organized into a coordinated network, builds meaningful partnerships with families and youth, and addresses their cultural and linguistic needs, in order to help them to function better at home, in school, in the community, and throughout life (Stroul et al., 2010). I reminisced about our high school students in New Jersey and the newly minted CRSs who worked so effectively with their families to help build a more congruent system of care.

Health care delivery has notoriously been directed to a single individual, with no ability to see or understand the tremendous influence of social determinants and social context. Expanding the system with a focus on "wellbeing" would require a dramatic pivot away from "Fix the acute problem in front of you." Planning and prevention require integration, coordination, and transparency. The health care system of America was broken, and Professor England's frustration, in 1995, rings loud and clear. In the ensuing 25 years, there are value-based pockets of health care excellence delivering efficient, high-quality, sustainable care. But the simple fact is that Black/Brown and poor families have worse health outcomes. The system needs to be repaired.

Esteemed Harvard professor, Robert D. Putnam, in his book *Our Kids: The American Dream in Crisis* (2015), explored the plight of America's children. After his visit to Port Clinton in Ohio, where he grew up, he found an economically failing region. When Professor Putnam was a child, factories boomed and the town had a strong sense of community. There was a robust societal belief that all of the children in the community were, in essence, all of "our children." Opportunities for kids born in the lower echelons to scale the socioeconomic ladder were abundant, he remarked. His 21st-century visit was heart-breaking. Juvenile delinquency rates were three times the national average; unwed births increased sharply to 40%, portending an increase in single parenting in the years ahead; and child poverty had skyrocketed. He described how the meaning of community drastically changed over the years—from aiding children and families to focusing on profit and adopting a "survival of the fittest" mentality (Putnam, 2015).

Professor Putnam stated that it was not simply the collapse of the working class because during this same time period he had witnessed the birth of a new upper class. What was important, he believed, at the time, was that everyone had an equal chance to climb the socioeconomic ladder; equality of opportunity and social mobility. This had disappeared.

Rebecca Vallas (associate director), along with Melissa Boteach (vice president of Half in Ten), both affiliated with the Poverty to Prosperity Program at the Center for American Progress, in 2014, reported that the Census Bureau revealed in its annual report that there was no significant improvement in the number of Americans living in poverty, post the economic recovery of 2008/2009. Low- and middle-income workers had seen no income growth over the past decade, leading many to believe that economic insecurity might be the new normal. Job creation, raising the minimum wage, increasing the earned income tax credit for childless workers, and supporting pay equity were among some of the steps they suggested might work to cut poverty, boost economic security, and expand the middle class (Vallas & Boteach, 2014). This sobering position with the ravages of COVID-19 will have worsened the situation.

Jason M. Breslow, digital editor at PBS Frontline, reported in 2012 that if we fail with our young people and their families, the cost to society is unthinkable (Breslow, 2012). He reported that the average high school dropout could expect to earn an annual income of $20,000 per year, according to the US Census Bureau; that is a full $10,000 less than a typical high school graduate, and $36,000 less than someone with a bachelor's degree. Additionally, 12% of high school dropouts are currently jobless, with 30% of them living in poverty. Among college graduates, joblessness is 4.1% with only 13.5% living in poverty (Breslow, 2012).

Anya Kamenetz, of NPR, in her publication, "From 'Dropout Crisis' to Record High, Dissecting the Graduation Rate," June 12, 2015, describes the state of dropping out. She quotes Robert Balfanz and Nettie Legters of Johns Hopkins University who singled out the nation's "dropout factories." At almost 1,000 high schools nationwide, they said your chances of graduating were no more than 50-50 (Kamenetz, 2015). The dropout rate disproportionately affects communities of color and low-income communities, and it was becoming a workforce issue. Sixty-three percent of jobs in the next decade would require some post-secondary education according to Sunny Deye (Kamenetz, 2015). The states had a legislative imperative to raise graduation rates. Kamenetz reported that Elaine Allensworth at the University of Chicago published work identifying early warning signs: attendance, behavior, and course performance.

Before 2005, paper records and attendance rolls were kept in metal file cabinets; technology eventually caught up to track individual students. In 2005, a task force was assembled to achieve a single, comparable, and accurate measure of graduation rates. The Adjusted Cohort Graduation Rate (ACGR) was adopted and put into practice (Kamenetz, 2015).

Good news arrived. The high school completion rate in America for 2014–2015 was approximately 81%, the highest percentage on record. And now the ACGR method appears to be working.

In the United States, it is estimated that each new graduate creates a net benefit of about $127,000 to the taxpayers over their lifetime. In 2012, it was further estimated that if the high school dropout rate was reduced by 700,000 it would create a net benefit to taxpayers of $90 billion for each year of success (Levin & Rouse, 2012).

One in ten male dropouts between the ages of 16 and 24 is either in prison or in juvenile detention. Juvenile incarceration decreases the likelihood of high school graduation by 13%. There is a direct correlation between a lack of high school education and incarceration (Choudry, 2018).

Dropping out predicts a significantly greater likelihood that a person will later become incarcerated. Forty-nine percent of children who have been in care will end up in the prison system (Snelle, 2015).

The New Zealand Government reported in a 2010 study that the average cost of maintaining a prisoner in New Zealand was $90,977 per year (Clayworth, 2012). Within New Zealand, 41% of all people convicted for the possession and/or use of illicit drugs in 2011 were between the ages of 17 and 24, which has significant repercussions on their future outcomes. Between 2007 and 2011, the New Zealand government spent $20,4709,500 on imprisoning people 25 and under for minor drug offenses (NZ Drug Foundation, 2013).

Conclusion

Reality does not necessarily cooperate with even our best theories. This chapter acknowledges the limitations of psychotherapy—even one as powerful as family therapy—with families overwhelmed by poverty and social upheaval. Life in poverty affects the functioning of the family system. The position of the CRS, working in tandem with a family therapy team, is an important enhancement to the system measuring outcomes and collecting data. The effectiveness of this role supports the IST theory of change: close the circle, increase coordination, and stabilize families by reducing their stress. Help the families reach for aspirational goals for their children—stay in high school and out of prison, so they can visualize prosperity for their futures.

In RBA, there is a value on population-based interventions. These expensive initiatives, like addressing community poverty or housing, are far beyond the reach of small non-profit organizations. However, the CRS, working with the microsystems of families, can successfully address education and employment, and lift the family to a new position and change the worrying poverty statistic that Breslow (2012) reported. This is a front-line, population-based concept, with small costs and big benefits. A better solution than waiting for this issue to be taken to scale with the poverty population.

8

BEYOND THEORY
OUTCOME-BASED SUPERVISION

Supervision is as old as guilds and professions. It is a time-honored tradition, universal, by which the clinical culture of one professional generation is transferred to the next. Or, some might say, it is the training of professionals by more experienced practitioners in formal feedback. Yet others might suggest that the supervisor and supervisee come together in a partnership for creating and tracking progress in families with problems. I am suggesting that supervision should be in accordance with the RBA tenet *Measure, measure, measure*. In the same way that RBA presents a new dimension in clinical work, it presents a similar valuable new perspective for supervision.

I was 26 years old, newly enrolled in the child psychiatry fellowship training, and there I was sitting in the innovatively designed Philadelphia Child Guidance Clinic (TV studio) treating a woman with a severe handwashing compulsion—up to 60 times a day. Her husband was sitting passively, looking stunned by the headlights of this unexplained chaos that had descended on his tidy life. Jay Haley, my supervisor, was behind

DOI: 10.4324/9781003161257-9

the one-way mirror watching and listening to my every move, twitch, and nuance. The wife explained that her hand washing compounded when she saw the man next door with his garden hose. This necessitated my taking a brief pause; I left the room and joined Jay behind the mirror, all the while forcing Sigmund from my thought processes.

Jay, a master strategist and the founder of Strategic Family Therapy, always supervised behind the mirror, never entering the therapy room. For Jay, therapy was an intellectual puzzle. He directed his supervisees to instruct the families with interventions to be carried out at home.

This 40-year-old married woman, a mother of two, who presented with this extreme hand-washing compulsion, was severely distressed. She had worked with a behaviorist prior to our meeting and was charting the number of times per day she washed her hands, as he suggested. This recommendation did not faze the problem and yet we asked her to continue this practice; it provided outcome data for our future interventions and minimized any criticism about his approach. Her compulsions had appeared when her husband's father died. He was then busy looking after his grieving mother every weekend for months, clearing out his parents' summer home, and leaving his wife alone with their two children.

Jay supervised me behind the mirror weekly; we were making little progress. His suggestion that the mother wear gloves to bed was reported as unsuccessful the following week. As a young supervisee, I was struggling with paradigms and there was no guidebook. I had no theory of change; I hoped one was looming in Jay's encyclopedic mind. I was totally reliant on the wisdom of my supervisor. I was discouraged, but Jay's mood was quite the opposite. He leaned back in his chair, with his mysterious bad leg up on the desk, and said in his laconic western voice, "You know Charles, we can crack this case tonight." I replied with some uncertainty. "Oh really?" I questioned, in a higher octave. Jay said, "Let's do the Devil's Pact."

It was the middle of a snowy Philadelphia winter and I was instructed to tell this couple that my wife and I would love to go somewhere warm, but we just didn't have the money. Further instructions from Jay were to boldly tell this increasingly skeptical couple, "I have the solution to your problem; I'm certain it will work. But before I explain the details of the plan, you must agree that you will follow it. Don't worry, it is not illegal and in no way unethical. I am confident it will be successful."

The session proceeded for 90 minutes; far exceeding the standard therapy time allocated for this room booking. There was probing and haggling and questioning this audacious promise. There were often moments of humor as they talked together and engaged in this surprising intervention. I witnessed this "ordeal" rendering the couple closer. They finally agreed and sat on the edge of their chairs awaiting the instruction. I then presented what Jay called "the Devil's Pact": "Every time you wash your hands, in the first week, it will cost you a dollar. In the second week, the price goes up to two dollars. The third week, you may choose three dollars per wash or alternatively, an exponential increase to six dollars per wash." They wisely chose the former. All the money would be paid for my trip to Jamaica. By the end of the session, the security guards had left the building and the temperature had taken a further drop. Walking to our respective homes in West Philly, Jay and I discussed the session. Jay was confident that the intervention would make a difference; I was less so.

The following week, as I walked into the consulting room with trepidation, the couple proudly presented their chart—the hand washing had almost disappeared. They reported that when they returned home the evening of the Devil's Pact, they had the biggest fight of their marriage. The husband promised his wife that he would reduce his time away from home, and their relationship appeared to have some sparks. The family only paid me a total of eight dollars; needless to say, no vacation that winter.

I called the family six months later for a follow-up and was told that the compulsive hand washing had fully disappeared. However, I was dismayed when the wife told me their sad news. The husband's mother had died unexpectedly of a cardiac arrest. She was in her middle sixties with no previous cardiac symptomatology. I cautiously wondered if our therapeutic jurisdiction should have expanded to include the grandmother; we had not appreciated that there might be consequences of her son's distancing, and she may have needed our help during this period.

In another one of my early cases, a four-year-old girl named Anna, described by her parents as a "monster," would frequently run out of the house and blindly stumble into the street. So dangerous, her parents had taken to padlocking her bedroom door at night to prevent a potential disaster. Salvador Minuchin, the second supervisor in my Fellowship year, walked into the room and "bummed" a cigarette from the father. He had an extraordinary ability to Join with everyone. He saw the therapist as an agent for change in the room through the Use of Self. He focused closely on a canon of techniques that the therapist would apply in response to family dynamics. I discovered that these techniques definitively transformed families in session.

Anna's father was a policeman, her mother a homemaker. She also had a sister, age two. The mother reported that Anna's father generally had more success in parenting both the girls. She said her husband acted as an authoritarian; he would "make" Anna do something if she was being difficult. The mother described herself as more passive, often compromising to let Anna have her way. She would often phrase her requests of Anna as questions, for example, "Go over there and play, okay?" Dr. Minuchin picked up on her tentative tone, and at one point asked the mother if she was afraid of her husband's way of handling their daughter. The mother said, "Yes, he's so big, and he can be a bit rough." The session proceeded with Minuchin gently helping the parents to agree on jointly moderating this little girl's behavior.

Sal invited the parents, along with myself, to the floor to play with the little children. The mother and the father were equally gentle and sweet with their daughters during this time. Minuchin complimented the father on his gentleness and this new behavior caught the attention of the mother. The parents presented a more united approach, and Anna became an adorable little girl; her "monster" behavior began to leave. Sal Minuchin, when inserting himself into a family by entering a room, always held surprises.

Jay Haley was a tactician and strategist. I trusted his judgment and followed his directives. He was so fully committed to his supervisees in the process of supervision that he left his honeymoon to supervise me when I had a family in crisis. Salvador Minuchin worked differently. He almost always entered the therapy room, and every intervention was an embodiment of one of his family therapy techniques. It felt magical, except that his model of treatment was transparent and the common language of techniques reproducible. These two supervisory sessions have been further discussed in books written by Haley (in *Problem-Solving Therapy*) and Minuchin and Fishman (in *Family Therapy Techniques*). This supervision cemented my belief in *mind in context*, and I had increased fidelity to this model. These therapeutic models and supervisory styles remained with me as I completed my Fellowship and moved to the positions of training and supervising others. Their personalities were strong; they lit up rooms and energized trainees. There was always a respect for families and a sensitivity to trainees that I gravitated toward. Upon reflection, I do think that, at times, even Haley and Minuchin were dazzled by the power and effectiveness of their models.

Haley supervised by teaching intervention strategies; Minuchin by teaching and modelling intervention techniques.

My supervision style and manner have waxed and waned over the years; there were minor adjustments as I traveled to different countries and supervised in non-English-speaking populations. But given what had been so deeply embedded by the supervision bestowed on me in my twenties, shaking that cloak of supervisory comfort did not come easily. The world was changing; "evidence" was becoming the quintessential buzz word and technology was rampaging. The recording studio in the Child Guidance Clinic, where therapy sessions were conducted, was considered by most "the state of the art," back in the day. I spent many dollars and recycled many cameras with fancy mountings, earnestly trying to recreate that studio in dozens of different work sites. Sourcing a reliable microphone did irritate. The one-way mirror, the critical tool of supervision, always rankled the budget people in governmental agencies when proposed; in my private clinic in New Jersey, we proudly boasted of one. It gnawed at my accountant.

My dusty files, hanging or parked in plastic sleeves and boxes of every size and shape holding labeled tapes, also of every size and shape, were resurrected as I began writing this book. I have managed to hold on to some of the machines that created the three-quarter-inch cassettes, the Hi8 ones, and the "new-fangled" digital ones. When I tell people that we worked with reel-to-reel recordings in the beginning, there is always disbelief. My iPhone of today is now my recording studio and "the cloud" holds the precious words and images; I no longer need a box. This is epic and helped to "down-size" the activity that all we baby boomers are talking about today.

I was not surprised when I uncovered an important historic document. Dr. Salvador Minuchin, supervising new family therapy trainees who were enrolled in a short, intensive training program, nearly 40 years earlier, was speaking to me again with clarity. I remember well the day this supervision was recorded; I used his tape often in those early years of my teaching. Somewhere along the way, I had the tape transcribed and there it was, in the hanging file. It harkens back to the period when he was introducing to the field the innovative concept that the therapist, working on a micro level, could be a well-honed instrument of change. These trainees were instructed to prepare segments of their therapy sessions where they were "stuck." These were early sessions of beginning therapists and they did report feeling quite stressed by the exercise. Alternatively, sometimes Sal would use what he called "roulette," where he would randomly stop one of their taped videos and begin commenting, thereby responding to an unplanned segment of the taped session. The genius of the therapy model has withstood all forms of modernization, unlike the recording machines. His clarity of thought washed over the trainees and hopefully to you, the reader.

Sal Minuchin Supervising Beginning Trainees Who Are "Stuck" (Transcribed, c. 1979)

Where possible, I have included some of the clinical information related to the cases.

Case One

Sarah is the identified patient (IP). She is 15 with various behavior problems. There are two other siblings, Tim (14) and Polly (six). The mother, Renee, is 37; the parents are divorced and the father lives out of town.

The trainee said that he was trying to reframe Sarah's problem as a family problem with the hope that the family would then agree to work on this. He stated that he had "failed at this."

Minuchin's responses:

1) *The therapist is trying to get Tim to be his co-therapist and by doing so, he is also saying to Mother, "I am making your son an evaluator of your behavior." Mother will*

resent this, and the boy should not join him in his collaboration. This is a dangerous activity, early in the game, although it is occasionally possible with adolescents. It is dangerous to enter into the hierarchy on the wrong side since this is subverting the cultural norm of the parents being on the top side of the hierarchy.

2) The therapist is too central. This makes it difficult to reframe because everything is directed to the therapist. The therapy needs more interaction in order to reframe what they are saying. The therapist is saying to the family, "I will solve your problem." By being so central, however, the family says, "Okay, solve our problem." The therapist hasn't lost the family; quite the opposite. He's got them, but now what? The family has accepted the therapist's centrality and he is stuck with a system in which all the weight is on him and he is drowning from it. The therapist is not mobilizing the family's capacity to bring about change for themselves.

3) The family has inducted the therapist by getting him to work for them. This happens very quickly in the session. The therapist fills the silence. The ball always finishes in his court; therefore, the therapist is too active. He is working inefficiently. He becomes a problem-solver. The silences always activate the therapist. There is probably an isomorph that the family brings to the therapy that there is someone in the system who enters with the problem-solving capacity. The therapist has been inducted into this position. The family has robbed him of his maneuverability.

4) The therapist needs to be less central to produce an Enactment. At the very least, he needs to provide a cognitive schema of possible alternatives and then ask the family which one they want to work on. The therapist has the capacity to be a strong leader. In fact, he's so good at this, this becomes a quicksand for him. The therapist could say things to this family like, "I don't know what way you get hooked into each other. It's a mystery; see if you can figure it out. Talk a little bit." Or, "Can you talk together?"

5) The therapist could use roulette with this family. Note, when the family begins to talk together, the therapist interrupts. One thing the therapist could do, à la Hoffman/ Haley techniques of family therapy, is give the family a task and then go behind the one-way mirror. (Lynn Hoffman).

Case Two

Lucy is the Identified patient, she is 14 and has truancy issues. This is an eight-member family: the grandmother, who is the legal guardian of the child, the grandfather, who is working at the time and crucial to the structure, Nancy is the mother, and Andrea, age 11, has a bad temper. All the other kids are reported to have "bad attitudes." The trainee reported that she had difficulties Joining.

1) Grandmother starts the session saying, "I am the boss and you need to teach her [my daughter] more." The therapist made a mistake in challenging the Grandmother. This is a problem in Joining since the culture gives legitimacy to Grandmother's leadership.

2) These people find it strange that the therapist asked the whole family to come when Andrea and Lucy are the problems. This family comes for a pill to cure them. The therapist must induct them to believe that he has a solution that's good for what they want.

3) The therapist needs an Enactment to see how the family responds. Then the therapist can say, "Here are a number of things I see are possible to change." The therapist tries to go to Lucy to talk. Grandmother says, "Another problem is, she doesn't talk." The therapist could say here, "You are absolutely right. She won't talk to me either." This will underline Grandmother's legitimate role as the leader, and then the therapist could say, "Can you get her to talk to you?" If Grandmother fails, then say, "Since Grandmother is unable, Mother, can you get your daughter to talk?" If Mother fails, say to Mother and Grandmother, "This is it, she doesn't talk to you." Then it becomes a challenge for the family to make her talk. The therapist can't make her talk against the family's power. She is too weak. The therapist cannot Join with the girl against the family, it's impossible. If Lucy Joins with the therapist, she will have an impossible time at home.

4) The therapist needs to convert the problem from one at home to something in the room. She needs to transform the symptom to make it happen—therefore the family needs to Enact it now. She can do this by finding a problem in the session—a lever in the family. It's always there—and use it.

5) The therapist must move from being the foreman to being a worker.

6) The therapist is weak compared with the power of the family. She must accept it and get others to work for her.

The session moves forward. The grandmother applies a punishment to Lucy. The therapist asks, "What do you want to happen?" The grandmother and the mother talk.

1) The therapist, at this point, should practice the art of being invisible, and look at her foot.

2) The therapist is too much of an accommodator. The therapist needs a punctuation guide, not of commas, but of periods and paragraphs. If she wants to accentuate grandmother/mother, she needs to de-accentuate grandmother/child and grandmother/therapist.

3) Good Joining allows the therapist to say to the family, "I'm telling you what to do and the two of you need to talk. I'm listening, but you talk." The therapist does this by Joining and un-Joining. If you Join all the time, then you are paralyzed—you're stuck. In this case, the therapist needs to activate people, especially Mother.

4) The therapist needs to make short statements that say, "I don't exist in this session except as a traffic cop." You've never seen a traffic cop talking to a driver.

5) In the mother/grandmother dyad, tension increases. The therapist enters, prompted by the increase in tension. Entering into the grandmother/mother triangle, the therapist is inducted. This availability of the therapist to enter to reduce the tension leaves her unable to think and do what she needs to do. In other words, if the process is at the level of proximity, you cannot get distance to think about the total picture. To the degree that the system controls you, you cannot think. You are too central.

6) What we are dealing with is an isomorphic pattern. Conflict between Mother and Grandmother and the entrance of a third person, albeit the therapist, the child, or Grandfather, is a repeated pattern of conflict. The therapist needs to change the pattern by focusing on one small issue. This concentration, then, allows the therapist to say to the family that it is isomorphic and represents the total picture. This helps to motivate the family.

7) In Joining, the family has a narrow view of the problem. The therapist can stress and not always support as a way of Joining. For example, the therapist can say, "You have a miserable life, do you want to change it?" Or, the therapist can Join by attacking, "What you are doing does not make sense."

8) This therapist is not Joining and Tracking well. There is a kind of boiler-plate quality to her interventions, especially in the last part. It is form-fitted to the family's content.

These transcribed notes are so classic Minuchin in his supervision. It is again based on process, on the belief that changing the interactional patterns and processes within the session, generalizing at home, and leading to better outcomes. The therapist learns in this supervision how to be a better agent of change by the Use of Self. Minuchin's razor-sharp perception of the therapist at work spots centrality, poor Joining, limited Enactments, and inability to be invisible. His analysis was always framed within the published techniques that he deemed so critical to working with families.

Literature Review

In recent years, marriage and family therapy (MFT) programs of various kinds have had varying success in integrating a research focus into their clinically oriented training structures. The traditional "scientist-practitioner" (Raimy, 1950) model, developed in the late 1940s, required psychology students to study research in the context of acquiring clinical skills (Frank, 1984). Although this model continues to work well in some cases (Hodgson et al., 2005), many family therapy (FT) programs (particularly at master's level) are moving to a less formal "research-informed" perspective, due to the scarcity of resources (time and means) to provide extensive research training (Karam & Sprenkle, 2010).

Although the current focus of (FT) supervision is stated to be on an "outcomes" approach (Rigazio-DiGilio, 2014, p. 622), the emphasis appears to remain on the knowledge and skills of the supervisee, as opposed to grounded data on how clients are progressing toward obtaining positive outcomes. Sandra Rigazio-DiGilio's contribution to The Wiley International Handbook of Clinical Supervision suggests that FT supervision should focus on "the conceptual, executive, and operational skills of a therapist to apply a systemic perspective" in their clinical work (Rigazio-DiGilio, 2014). Indeed, in-vogue models of FT supervision share a common focus on the supervisor–supervisee relationship and provide lengthy frameworks through which supervisors can develop a good understanding of their supervisees (Morgan & Sprenkle, 2007; Breunlin et al., 2011; Todd & Storm, 2014). While a focus on the therapist's understanding and world view, and their functioning in a relationship with the supervisor, is undoubtedly important, I hold that the field of family therapy would benefit from a shift in its supervision focus more toward clients' outcomes and the measures that indicate whether an intervention is actually working. Importantly, the idea of a relationship might be better served to shift to a partnership model whereby each is bearing responsibility for outcomes.

In developing their Dyadic Supervision Evaluation (DSE) Assessment tool, Avila and colleagues (2016) conducted an exploratory factor analysis of 50 possible competencies for FT trainees and supervisors. Although all of these competencies have face validity, none of the competencies were explicitly focused on client outcomes. Similarly, Wallace and Cooper (2015) identified 11 key dimensions to be considered in the construction of new family supervision tools; none of them were client outcomes. These tools aim to be "empirically validated" (Avila et al., 2016, p. 284), however, I wonder how this can be so if there is no evidence linking any of these competencies with objective client outcome measures.

It seems that family therapists may not see supervision as a process to enhance a therapist's ability to produce better outcomes for their clients. Sixteen family therapists in northern Europe formed a reflective research forum that spanned two years in order to articulate practical guidelines for FT supervision. They concluded that the most important elements of FT supervision were: 1) an agreed contract; 2) flexibility in format; 3) to explore the content of sessions; and 4) for the supervisor to take responsibility for process and dilemmas (Flåm, 2016). Responsibility was focused on process and again no mention of outcomes.

Although the prevalence of outcome-focused RCTs has steadily increased in the FT literature, the field has been wary of their validity, given the natural diversity of clinical circumstances in which family therapists operate (Sexton et al., 2008). Sexton and colleagues (2008, p. 392) concluded that moving toward more "diverse research methods" will be a key move for the field moving forward.

Within the field of FT, however, there are some models that more explicitly focus on client outcomes, and this extends to their supervisory practices. For example, within multisystemic therapy's (MST) supervisory practice, a supervisor's focus remains squarely on the outcomes of the client (Karamat Ali & Bachicha, 2012). Research on the effectiveness of this stance is promising. One study examined the relationship between an MST supervisor's adherence to the protocol and young clients' behavior and functioning one year after treatment had concluded. Greater adherence to the structure and process of MST supervision during the treatment protocol predicted positive shifts in youth behavior in the 12-months follow-up (Schoenwald et al., 2009). It seems that if there is a supervision protocol in place that focuses on client outcomes, and supervisors adhere closely to it, there is an observable, long-term benefit in terms of client wellbeing.

C.E. Watkins published in 2011 about thirty years of research on whether supervision contributes to patient outcomes. "If we cannot show that supervision affects patient outcome, then how can we justify supervision?" The research established that supervision positively impacts the supervisee across various domains yet there appears to be an ongoing paucity of research towards what has been referred to as the "acid test" (Watkins, 2011)

IST/RBA Supervision Model

My historical supervision from Haley and Minuchin remained with me for many years. Results-based accountability, however, abruptly challenged my well-honed ideas and shifted my orientation. A performance-based model focused my supervision to its rightful jurisdiction—the outcomes precinct, opening up the supervisory process to feedback loops and targeting what works, with the understanding that the supervisor and supervisee have equal responsibility.

I am presenting a supervisory system intended to be bring mastery. I see this system applicable to the family therapist or trainee wherever they might be working/studying. The Clinician's Mastery Report was developed to help guide the clinician toward achieving those skills essential for successful outcomes. The report includes protocols for common mental health conditions, the use of the Homeostatic Maintainer Searchlight, the IST Triangulation and Single Parent Scales. There is a section, the Alphabet of Skills, that requires fidelity to the structural family therapy model found in the book on 'technique.' Each treatment protocol and skill is detailed for the trainee/therapist using a Likert scale to lead their way.

TERMS OF REFERENCE (IS ANYONE BETTER OFF?)

The terms of reference have been developed for the supervisee and supervisor. To accomplish shared goals, the purpose and structures have been detailed. Working together in partnership, they detail authority and delegate responsibilities.

1) Supervisor and supervisee agree to the theory of change based on IST/RBA framework to avoid potential conflicts with other supervisors and remove any hints of triangulation;

2) Transformation will be focused on the contemporary system;

3) The Clinical Scorecard will be developed and utilized for each client providing observed grounded data for the clinician and supervisee;

4) The targets that are established on the Clinical Score Care determine the clinician's and the team's performance. Achieving the target is the outcome;

5) The supervision partnership will be reviewed with systematic periodicity, e.g., quarterly for outcome: The Turning the Curve tool will provide a snapshot of progress for the partners. The slope provides final outcome data for the treatment of the case;

6) The supervisory sessions will take many forms and be tailored to the clinician's workplace. In addition, the supervisor, when live supervising will refer to the Alphabet of Skills Scale, learning style, and experience;

7) The supervisee will be encouraged to develop a self-learning approach to supervision whereby he/she will advise the supervisor of the areas needing attention. When supervisees become reflective about the teaching and learning process, they strengthen their own capacity. This will be confirmed by the Clinician's Mastery Report. This can take many forms, tailored to the clinician's workplace, learning style, and experience;

8) The supervisor's skills will be measured against the therapist's mastery and outcomes in the Clinician's Mastery Report;

9) The duration of supervisory engagement will be based on the supervisees' outcomes of their practice and their Clinical Mastery Report;

10) Outcomes of the treatment of patients'/clients' problems will contribute to the published evidence.

SUPERVISORY METHODS

- Supervisor provides strategic advice to the clinician throughout the course of the treatment;
- Supervisor teaches and assesses the clinician's 'Use of Self' by using the Alphabet of Skills (developed from Family Therapy

Techniques); the supervisor reviews the video tapes or directly observes the therapy sessions;

- Supervisor teaches and evaluates the Homeostatic Maintainer Searchlight;
- Supervisor teaches and evaluates the clinician's use of the Triangulation and Single Parent's Scales;
- Supervisor teaches and evaluates mastery of treatment of common mental health conditions: psychosomatic family (AN, BN, COE), school avoidance, and conduct disorder;
- Supervisor assesses and marks the Clinician's Mastery Report, reflecting progress in all the above areas. The Turning the Curve tool is used to track the clinician's outcomes and all of the measures nominated in the Mastery Report;
- Under supervision, the therapist becomes a local clinical scientist. The Curve becomes the accepted standard of reporting outcomes and therefore the results are easily applied to basic efficacy studies. The clinician practices and reports real-world conditions and outcomes, adding to the plethora of published research.
- Supervisor models and teaches reflective process.

Note: The Clinician's Mastery Report and the Reflection Tool are found in the Appendix.

Conclusion

Models of supervision have changed over the years from process notes to the dreaded ghostly call from behind the one-way mirror. Today, the one-way mirror may be replaced by live streaming. Regardless of the technology, adding measurements, the heart of science, to a supervisory method, will advance clinical performance. *Yes, everybody is better off!*

Note: A review of the accountable, measurable supervisory schema can be found in the Appendix.

9

PATTERNS THAT CONNECT

The goal of this book is to help you on the road to mastery. We are in the business of excellent outcomes.

I use the concept of isomorphism to create a solid place for the master clinician to stand on, to observe and transform their work with underlying connecting patterns of their clients, the families. Mathematicians use the word isomorphism to describe a structure-g mapping between two structures of the same type. In today's family therapy literature, it is most commonly used to describe parallel processes between the therapist and the supervisor. It's even used to describe transference!

The word "isomorphism" is derived from the Ancient Greek: ἴσος (isos, equal) and μορφή (morphe, form or shape). It is an interactional pattern that is formed and has the capacity to replicate in different contexts; its tenacious power can bring therapists to their knees. The skill to identify and modify these patterns is the *sine qua non* of a master therapist. Recurring themes in the family fugue ideally sing out to the clinician. The pitches may change as the harmonic context changes, but the connecting

DOI: 10.4324/9781003161257-10

relationships remain the same. Families organized around fugue themes (or isomorphs) can be expected to carry over behaviors from the family context to other contexts and probably to future generations.

The family member can be viewed as a member of an orchestra, playing the tuba, practicing in his or her apartment on a Saturday morning. If we were listening upstairs, we would hear silence, then the tuba notes, then more silence. In the musician's head, the entire orchestra is being heard. But we neighbors hear only the tuba-staccato, loud and seemingly random. The tuba sounds ridiculous because the musician and the neighbors are responding to the rules of different systems. As I sit over my coffee, listening to the tubist practice, I long for the orchestra. But for the tuba player, conforming to a system whose rules are written on the score and played in his or her head, the constraints are different, and resoundingly real.

A full symphony is appreciated by a therapist when all the family members are assembled and interacting. The isomorphs are revealed. Each member's behavior is complementary to the other. Minuchin called this "the family dance." In well-functioning families there is great latitude, a constant process of adaptation. In troubled families, there seems to be an inflexibility that encourages repetition and the same dance steps.

The opening sentence of Leo Tolstoy's *Anna Karenina* is, "All happy families are alike; each unhappy family is unhappy in its own way." Tolstoy was a great novelist but not a family therapist. From my perspective, it's the other way around: happy families have great creativity and flexibility. Unhappy ones follow stereotypical patterns, manifesting relatively few isomorphic patterns that get used and reused in a myriad of contexts. They certainly don't mean to do that; the pesky contextual demands 'rev' up the automaticity and override free will.

My Sunday afternoon family therapy supervision, a *hui* (gathering, a Māori word), was initiated by friends and colleagues in New Zealand. It is a 90-minute Zoom tutorial that now includes child psychiatrists, psychologists, and counselors from New Zealand, Australia, Hawaii, and the US mainland. Some are early in their training and others are further along. All are keenly interested in family therapy. A heavy dose of case discussion is bolstered with theoretical didactics. There is no direct observation of their clinical work or video tape review, unless I am using my tapes. My role is to consult on their cases, 'the ones that keep them up at night.' With such wide diversity of the membership, I reasoned that the family therapy focus required a framework for each participant to anchor their understanding. Learning family therapy can sometimes be a great challenge for some, especially if it comes later in their training. I have seen this during my decades of teaching and supervising. Many members are working in different milieus with conflicting treatment models; they roam the hallways of their institutions, sometimes frustrated. My responsibility was to alleviate confusion. I do not assume responsibility for their cases in the same partnership way that my supervision model has been explained.

The hui is the protected time for clinicians to cross over and become family therapists. Adopt the concepts and language and engage safely in robust discussion. I introduced isomorphism, a grounded perspective. The simplicity of "Lift the hood (or bonnet) and examine the family's motor" was the rallying cry for assessment. Strike the isomorphic pattern and persist; this was the interventional intention; the framework for shifting nonfamily therapists in the world of families. Be warned, historical deflections of your patients or families may derail your progress.

Since my college days, I have been interested in the concept of deep structures that underlie the phenomenology of the human experience. I did mention this to Salvador Minuchin when we first met. The structural anthropologist, Claude Lévi-Strauss (1962), believed that culture was like a language, with hidden rules that govern behavior. He said this was what made cultures unique. The participants accommodate but cannot articulate the rules. It is therefore up to us to identify them. He analyzed these structural relations among their elements and introduced the commonality of structures. I speculate that Strauss's hidden rules, the deep structures, are the isomorphic patterns.

In Gregory Bateson's (2002) writings, he described people, relationships, and events as looking for coherence, "patterns that connect." The notion of interactional patterns of consequence was his holistic paradigm that created the basis of family therapy; the terra firma where isomorphs reside.

An emphasis on the family system as a whole is where the entire orchestra is heard. Homeostasis glues the musicians together, but their music is discordant. Homeostasis keeps the family systems stuck. This is the moment when you search for isomorphs, the ability to penetrate and make a difference.

Isomorphism, according to Koltz et al. (2012), is inter-relational and believed to have originated in the field of family therapy as a systemic counterpart to parallel process. While isomorphism has been used interchangeably with the term parallel process, it is believed to be quite different with regard to focus (Koltz et al., 2012). Parallel process is intrapsychic, according to Bradley and Gould (2001, cited in Koltz et al., 2012). Isomorphism is inter-relational and presents itself as replicating structural patterns between counseling and supervision (White & Russell, 1997, cited in Koltz et al., 2012). Blake Edwards (2015), in discussing isomorphism as intervention, says it is about intentionality as a therapist in cultivating emotional-relational transparency oriented toward therapeutic intimacy. The origins of parallel process are in the psychoanalytic concepts of transference and countertransference, according to Marie Sumerel (1994). Rynes et al. (2014) believe that isomorphism, or parallel process, occurs in family therapy when patterns of therapist–client interaction replicate problematic interactional patterns within the family.

The original work in family therapy was steeped in isomorphism. The patterns were observable, giving scientific credence to predictability. A psychosomatic family with psychosomatic interactional patterns, when stressed, would manifest medical complaints. Isomorphism, for some, may conceptualize the relationship between supervisor and supervisee. I, and the founders of structural therapy such as Braulio Montalvo use it differently; it is a way for a clinician to be more effective in treating families (personal communication, 1987). They observe the problematic patterns (isomorphs) and intervene. The effectiveness of supervision is to gauge the outcomes the supervisees achieve with their families, not their relationship with me.

The skill of locating isomorphic patterns provides opportunities for the clinician to intervene with confidence. The clinician walks into the therapy room with a prepared list of isomorphs, a mental database, knowing that the family will most likely manifest one or more of these patterns.

Isomorphs are vibrant. They guide clinicians. Therapy is planned and shaped on the basis of an isomorph. The currency of conversation in my

Sunday Afternoon Supervision was the list of common isomorphs. When these clinicians prepare to intervene with their families in treatment, they were instructed to look for their dysfunctional patterns. Their motors were running but clearly needed adjustments. Isomorphs are simple, focused, and the first step toward planning treatment. In my book with Minuchin, *Family Therapy Techniques* (1981), we urged clinicians to train for "spontaneity." Studying and using these isomorphic patterns is an important step toward "informed spontaneity" and creating a well-prepared mind.

Isomorphic Patterns: These Patterns Emerge within Families and Broader Systems

1) Enmeshment—blurring boundaries between family members;
2) Psychosomatic family—five characteristics are described in-depth in this book: enmeshment, conflict avoidance, overprotectiveness, rigidity, and triangulation;
3) Disengaged family—emotionally detached;
4) Disrupted hierarchy;
5) Triangulating family system;
6) Conflict avoidant family;
7) Complementary and symmetrical sequences;
8) Chaotic family system;
9) Rigid system.

The structural model of family therapy opened the door to isomorphs; we encapsulated the concept when conducting family therapy. They are not intellectual constructs, like diagnoses, but patterns that can be described and transformed. When detected, the clinician will intervene, and shift the family to a more coherent pattern in real time. They do predict the behavior of the system and even the functionality.

In keeping with RBA, I suggested to the clinicians that they must track the effectiveness of intervening with the isomorphic patterns. Setting targets and readjusting to achieve the stated goals; reaching successful outcomes.

What follows are clinical cases that were discussed, (transcribed conversations) illustrating isomorphs in action. Many are cases presented by members of the Sunday group; others come from different professional contexts. The clinicians and details around the case presentations have been anonymized.

Case One: The Isomorph Tutorial

The message to the group was simple: Locate the isomorphic pattern that needs to be transformed. Piggyback the relevant content presented by the families onto their patterns.

> *HCF: This is a tape of an anorectic woman who had been starving herself for 20 years. She was 42 years old, married with two children, ages 11 and 15. This is the second session with her parents. When she called me initially for an appointment, I asked her, "Tell me a little bit about your family." And she said, "My parents are driving me crazy." During the first session, a major issue came up; it was their Sunday morning brunches together. D and her husband would make brunch for her parents, but her parents would never tell them what time they would arrive at the house. D and her husband would never ask, and they said they felt like hostages. They had never challenged the parents about their erratic arrival times.*

Commentary: This is a psychosomatic family. Interestingly, D's childhood had exactly the same experience with her grandparents' visits to her family home. .

All interventions in the session are directed to the psychosomatic process pattern. When I walked into the room and asked, "How is everybody?" The grandparents said, "Ok," the husband said nothing, and D said, "Everyone's ok, except for me." I see this as indicative of how her symptoms are the focus of the family and defusing the tension and conflict within the session. I go directly to the conflict avoidance pattern (isomorph), it is a much easier handle for creating change than the other psychosomatic characteristics. If the conflict is manifested and resolved, then the other characteristics of the psychosomatic pattern ameliorate.

> D: Great, uh-huh, except for me! I don't think this is very easy, it isn't easy for me.
> HCF: How come?

Commentary: She is diffusing the tension by presenting herself as having a problem. She has done this for 20 years with her anorexia.

> D: This is the worst thing I have ever done!

Commentary: This woman has given birth to two children and raised them into adolescents, and the most difficult thing she has done is see a therapist (me) with her parents. This is one conflict-avoidant system!

> HCF: It is?
>
> D: Yes. I wish it could be as simple as that. I learned last week that my father had been involved in breaking up an important relationship when I was in college.
>
> HCF: Let's talk about Sunday mornings. [Looking at D, I suggest that she and her husband need to talk directly to her parents to change the visits so they are more to her liking.]

Commentary: I directly address the pattern of conflict avoidance. I do not discuss the historical deflection about the important relationship when she was in college.tempting though it may be, it would not lead to a structural change. D, with the help of her husband, will need to challenge the chronic pattern of the Sunday brunches. The grandparents' reaction to discussing this conflict in the session the previous week, when they had been gently challenged, was telling. Her father had said, "If you feel that way about it, to hell with you." He infers that it is "my way or the highway"; there is no discussion to be had. That is the rigidity of the system. Like all families, this family is imperfect, but the father rejects this notion. These characteristics of the psychosomatic model maintain the problem. We cannot directly access every characteristic but we can access the system's allergy to confronting one another.

> D's father: I miss my grandchildren.
>
> D: Well, you could come over.

Commentary: D's father brings out the big guns: guilt. And D capitulates, avoiding the conflict.

HCF: B, you really miss your grandchildren a lot? [I'm increasing the conflict by adding Intensity.]

D's father: Oh, I see them. They miss me more than I miss them.

Commentary: Again, he adds the guilt; I assume he is trying to get his daughter to relent. This is likely what he has done in the past. With my supporting D, I am hopeful that she will roll up her sleeves, and advocate for herself. I push for the conflict; the very thing that the family avoids. This is the counter-isomorph for the conflict-avoiding psychosomatic family.

HCF: Good, that's fine. But, go ahead, talk more about how you miss the Sundays?

D's father: Oh, you mean me? Miss them?

D's mother: I think, just the truth is that, we said...

D: I didn't say it.

D's mother: You said we should come at 12:30 instead of 2:00.

D's father [to his wife]: And then you cut your finger off because...

D: Oh, you cut your finger because we said 12:30 when you were chopping the mushrooms?

D's mother: Because, ok, I'll tell you what, because I know that he gets aggravated. I know that it bothers him [her husband].

Commentary: Here is triangulation, how D is caught between her parents. What I believe might be curative for this system, at this point, is to continue to provoke the conflict and support toward resolution.

D: I try to make peace and I don't do it very well.

D's mother: I just feel that it's all so perpetual.

D: I have always done that, you have spent every Sunday in that house, your whole life, and I just felt...

Commentary: So, the system is very rigid.

HCF: It's just like you spent your Sundays at your parents' house.

D: Every Sunday of my entire life was spent there.

D's mother: When you cut your finger, it's a big thing, believe me. It's important! (She laughs and looks to me, looking at confirmation that her daughter was wrong. I ignore her attempt.)

HCF: Let's discuss a conflict that you avoided this week?

D: We didn't have one this week. I don't have conflicts anymore.

HCF: It seems to me, that everybody in your family is a conflict avoider.

D: "Ignore it and it will go away."

HCF: Everybody seems to thrive on it.

D: Well, what happens when you avoid conflict all the time?

HCF: Things don't change. And to the extent that things don't change, you focus on not eating, on the anorexia. Talk to your parents about it, because...

D's mother: ...if anything, for years I've been aware, trying not to upset you in any way... trying to avoid, I would make sure that I never offered advice unless you said, "Mother, what do you think of this?" I was conscious of the fact that, "I better not, I'll wait 'til she asks, I don't want to upset her."

HCF: *What about that, are there areas where you think your relationship needs to change? Are there things that D does that bother you? Things you've been putting in cold storage all these years?*

D's mother: Well, sure. I would like her to eat. Now, not even talking about other stuff.

D: [laughs] I think that might be the basis for the whole thing. By the end of the session, she forthrightly challenges her parents, insisting that Sunday visits are revised.

Commentary: This is a case that I presented in-depth in my book Enduring Change in Eating Disorders: Interventions with Long-Term Results (2004). With an eight-month treatment focusing entirely on transforming the patterns of the psychosomatic family, the problem ceased. A two-year follow-up and she was doing fine; D had gained 50 pounds and was happy in her marriage. Twenty years after the treatment, the anorexia had not recurred.

Case Two: Occam's Razor

C: Clinician-This is a client who I saw regularly ten years ago when he was a CEO in New York. He has come back to see me. He's just bought a house, with his second wife, and they have a young child. They appear to be a well-functioning family system. He has four children with his ex-wife.

When back in his country, he was caught off guard when his father asked, "Will you come and help me take some things out of the boat?" This triggered a memory. "I'm not going into that boat; that's where that teenager sexually abused me." He remembered he was about 10; he had some vague memories of an older boy, 18, masturbating in front of him and asking him to pull his pants down. His father persisted and asked him again if he would go to the boat, he said he felt dismissed. "Dad, I was sexually abused in that boat."

This is the point when our therapy restarted. We did some trauma work and some somatic experiencing. The sexual abuse memories started coming back and he was having a lot of emotion. He subsequently went to the police and reported the incident. The police told him that the guy was a well-known pedophile; they wanted to know if there were others. "Oh yeah, I remember one boy." He asked the police not to contact him; he would rather do it.

The day after our session he contacted the man. "I want to talk to you about something, he said". The man said, "It happened, didn't it?" Then they both burst into tears and shared their stories. More memories emerged. There was confusion about his sexual orientation. Strong super-ego attacks, and then memories about his whole childhood. He realized that both his parents were alcoholics. When his mom was breastfeeding, she would have a glass of wine in one hand, and a cigarette in the other.

HCF: *How does he know?*

N: This was the family story; everyone thought it really funny. He told me they each drank about two bottles of wine a night, their whole life, so basically, "I've grown up in an alcoholic family."

He realized he's had suicidal thoughts his whole life. Going to bed very late at night because that's when his suicidal thoughts came on; self-medicating, and now he's decided not to drink. He's just staying with the emotions and feelings. We continue doing the trauma work and he's feeling a lot more regulated; much better. Now his whole family looks totally different, they're not the family he thought they were.

HCF: *His family of origin?*

N: Yes, his family of origin.

HCF: *So why did he come to see you?*

N: He'd just finished this big piece of work in New York and was feeling anxious; had apathy. Before that he was fine. He had anxiety, a bit of depression, re-adjusting to his new life. Then came the flood of memories, triggered by his father saying, "Will you come and help me clear the boat?"

He described three sets of academic parents, and they would all socialize and drink together and the eldest boy would look after all the kids. He remembers several times telling his parents he didn't want to go and stay with this babysitter, but they didn't hear him. So I'd be really interested from a family therapy point of view, how to treat this man.

HCF: I want to know about his marriages.

N: His first marriage?

HCF: Is there strife with his first wife and children from that marriage?

N: No.

HCF: Regarding his present marriage, the contemporary family system, are he and his wife doing well together?

N: Very good marriage. But that's because years ago in the first marriage, it was really not good. His wife had anorexia, she was very like his mother, not attached to the children.

HCF: Ok.

N: So he's been married now with this woman for twelve years and they have an amazing relationship. From what I can see, from what he says, she adores him, he adores her.

HCF: What is the pain that he's feeling?

N: Um, so the pain was after the end of this job and not quite knowing, coming back to his country of origin and just wanting to kind of reconnect.

HCF: So, let's look at it differently.

N: ...and then depression and anxiety. Yep. But I think it's because of this whole sexual abuse. That's how it looks from my perspective; it's all embedded in the context of his family and the alcoholism and...

HCF: I'm striving for us to look at the contemporary system and find some real-time grounded data. He leaves this business, ideally very successfully?

Commentary: There is an avalanche of history; to bring about change, we must find what will transform this system.

N: Not as successfully as he thought he would.

HCF: *He changes to a new context and he's lost. I've seen this before. It's a tremendous relief selling your business, but then the question is, what do you do. It's been the focus of your life. It is the "who am I" question.*

N: Yeah. And he didn't get the payout he wanted. He thought he'd be independently wealthy.

HCF: *So, there you go.*

N: It was a disappointing exit.

HCF: *So he needs to get another job?.*

N: He's got no pressure on him because his wife has a very good new job.

HCF: *They're both in transition—him from his job, her from her new job.*

N: Yes. Although at the moment he's quite happy not to work and just to come back to himself.

HCF: *But I thought you said he's adrift.*

N: He's still adrift, yeah.

HCF: *So the question is, how does he find a place in his new community. Do you see his wife?*

N: Not individually. I've spoken to her because I was concerned about him. I have spoken to his brother also.

HCF: *The wizened clinician that I am, when people tell me they have a happy marriage, I need to know more. Many of the problems are based in the marriage, our key relationship.*

N: Yeah. But I can assure you, Charles, I mean, unless I'm blind...

HCF: *Have you seen them together?*

N: Yeah, um, I've seen them twice together. They look like they have an amazing relationship. I think he's very emotionally available, she's very emotionally available, they're very connected. As far as I can see he's very close with his brother...

HCF: I think that this can be a difficult transition, moving and leaving your job but I suspect there is more strife in his life, judging from the suicidal ideation. So then the question is, what are some of the contemporary forces of instability. I mean, he comes to see you because he has some psychological distress. For example, how often does he talk to his father?

N: Um, he was estranged and distant from his parents. But since we worked together ten years ago he seems to be a lot closer. He says when he lived in New York his parents wouldn't visit. It was out of their way, so it was always him making the effort to see them; "Can I bring the kids to the airport so they can see you?" The parents never really made much effort with the kids (grandchildren)...

HCF: It may well be that the emotional distance and conflict remain.

N: Although he says in the last ten years there isn't any, they've been very close and affectionate with his parents.

HCF: Alright. I'm interested in what's going on now.

N: He has confronted his parents. He told them details about the sexual abuse, that he's informed the police. He told them he'd met this other boy (man), and the first comment the father said was, "Oh, you're not putting ideas in each other's heads, are you?"

Commentary: So again, the parents have been quite ineffectual, even rejecting in responding to their son's pain. Is this the contextual split that is generating his stress? He tells his parents, "I love you," giving them a hug, and they're not spontaneous in terms of giving him a hug back. They're creating distance from the whole thing. They do not know how to respond.

N: But he now understands. His new realization is they don't have the capacity, and so he's letting go of the expectation for them to respond in the way he would like them to. That's what he's saying.

HCF: From a therapeutic point of view, I wouldn't give him that alibi. I would say to him, "It sounds like your parents are questioning and rejecting your concerns." If he tells his parents something that's really upsetting him, they say in essence, "It's all in your head." They're busy gaslighting.

N: Yeah, that's what they're doing. So the only thing then would be to bring everyone together for family therapy; bring the parents in?

HCF: *This is a conflict-avoiding family.*

N: Probably no conflict; no conflict between the parents, even though the mother is very controlling and highly, highly intelligent. The father's very passive.

HCF: *I would challenge them to work it out? Deal with the conflict. It may be the "stiff upper lip" kind of thing. People will never tell you what they think. But they tell the next person.*

N: That's interesting you say that, because this client never told me before that he always had suicidal ideation.

HCF: *It's a poignant moment when he tells his dad about this sexual abuse and his dad blames him.*

N: Yeah. Yeah. Or they've just totally ignored it, not taken it in.

HCF: *It's their avoidance and seemingly systemic rigidity. The other prevailing isomorph is the parents are disengaged from their son. Hopefully, in the process of addressing the conflict avoidance, the family will become closer.*

N: It is conflict avoidance, to not talk about it, to not want to know?

HCF: *Yes. Bring the family in and help them work it out. His symptoms will likely remit.*

Commentary: As I discussed in Chapter 4, transform the contemporary system and you tend to ameliorate the presenting problems. Back to Occam's razor, the simplest explanation is always preferable. He advocated for transparent data, which is what I was searching for—and we found it when we focused on the man's relationship with his father and mother.

The isomorph is disengaged. The man and his parents, especially his father, have chronically managed this upsetting experience in their son's life by distancing—avoiding. He portends to lower his expectations for his parents, but the fact is, he has been bereft and suicidal many times.

Addendum

My model focuses on the contemporary system; with PTSD, a disorder rooted in the past, you may find symptom presentation waxes and wanes on the basis of the immediate social pressures.

Many years ago, I was invited to present at a veterans' conference. In preparation, I interviewed a number of veterans who were being treated for PTSD. One of the veterans told me the following: he worked at the post office and said that his supervisor did not trust him and would follow him occasionally on his postal routes; his brother-in-law had a psychosis and was threatening him with a gun-he was back in the rice paddies of Vietnam. He said that the PTSD only resurfaced after these pressures emerged.

I discussed this idea with a woman who reported having severe PTSD after serving in Iraq. She said that was her experience, symptoms waxed and waned in the context of contemporary pressures e.g, leaving her abusive husband.

The treatment of PTSD is not my area of expertise but immediate social pressures do need to be examined and addressed.

Case Three: The Hermit

HCF: I'm interested in the dynamics of family systems, meat and potatoes stuff. Let me give you an example. A young man, 26 years old, called for an appointment, "I'm suffering from compulsive over-eating." The next day, he did not show up. A few months later, his mother called, "Did you see my son in therapy?" "No, he did not show up." "He's been sending me your bills to reimburse him." "Sorry, I've never seen him or sent him a bill."

A month later, she called for an appointment; they arrived together, along with the uncle. He was medium stature and obese, bloated. He had little to show for his 26 years—had not completed high school and had never held a job; he had few friends and no skills. He lived primarily in his childhood bedroom. He appeared to have no idea of the extreme developmental danger he was in.

N: Obviously the parents are tolerating it if he's 26.

HCF: No, just the mother. The father is long gone; he is a professor living in another country. The mother has organized countless therapists for him but nothing has changed. The terms of reference were clear: help this young man start a life.

I supported and challenged the mother to get him "unstuck." I could have spent a thousand years, but I would never have the leverage to do it. After two months, he snagged a volunteer job, a lifetime first. Six months later, with an ultimatum from his generous mother, he found a place to live. He was ticking along; his obesity remained. Sadly, the volunteer position was lost during COVID and he was again trapped; doing nothing. Why did he not budge?

N: It's about his mother, his relationship with his mother...

HCF: His mother gives him no money. His general practitioner had organized a benefit based on some medical condition, further de-incentivizing him. I reasoned that a dose of poverty might help him recognize his developmental danger. He appeared to have scant ideas that his mother would die before him—leaving him desperately poor. Six months later, as the world returned to normal, he finally succeeded in achieving a full driver's license. He walked into the Work and Income Office and terminated his benefit, on his own, with a bit of urging from the mother. He landed a full-time job delivering pizzas, using his mother's car.

Commentary: The prevailing isomorph is enmeshment. At critical developmental stages in this man's life, his mother capitulated. He wanted to quit high school; he said the teachers did not like him. Tackling a teenager's insecurities was too difficult. It threatened her closeness to him; it was easier to let him leave school and sleep upstairs.

With the isomorph in mind, I direct the therapy to create every opportunity where mother and son can increase their distance: work, place of residence, driving, and living with a roommate. His libido is finally awake and he is interested in dating; hopefully creating a family of his own.

Case Four: Cannabis Girl

T: A 17-year-old girl was referred to me from The Medical Center; I've seen the family twice. She has been hospitalized five times for cannabinoid hyperemesis. The parents discovered for the first time that she's been smoking marijuana every day for about a year and a half to two years. They haven't been able to get her to commit to any follow-up after her previous hospitalization so they're trying something new by coming to me. The parents are together, the mom is a receptionist, the dad works in the commercial plumbing industry.

The three came to the first appointment together. They did mention that they had completed some marital counseling. The mom got a therapist for herself because of the worry about the recurrent hospitalizations of her daughter. She was having high anxiety and then she and her husband started going to the therapist together. They said it's helped their communication.

They searched their daughter's room after the second hospitalization, when they were told about her marijuana use. Her dad found the drugs and got rid of them. Now they're afraid to search her room again; well, the mom's afraid, she doesn't want to break her daughter's trust. The girl's failing school. She barely passed the last year. The dad says he'd be happy if she just gets Ds, he just wants her to pass her classes. She is going into her senior year, final year. There is money set aside for her from a trust to go to college, and she doesn't know if she wants to do that. It's been a huge source of stress. She feels tremendous pressure to use the money.

She's had some suicidal thoughts, hasn't really acted on them. She appears depressed and the parents wonder about medications, but are open to other things as well.

When I next see them all together, we will talk about next steps. I'm not sure what the dynamics are or what my target should be. And I think of the leverage (intensity): she's failing out of school, or near failing, and she has suicidal thoughts. It would be great to get everyone's input.

B: Well, I have a couple of questions. She's 16 or 17?

T: 17.

HCF: Let's think more simply. What is the problem? This spoilt little girl isn't doing any homework, she's breaking the law, and the mother's concerned about upsetting her and breaking her trust. She's on a downward trajectory. All she needs is a baby next year.

She is treated like a vulnerable child. Was she sick as an infant or something like that? Is she an only child?

T: No, she has an older sister who is in college.

HCF: Right. So they tiptoe around this kid.

B: Why do they do that?

HCF: You may get an answer, but it will likely offer little help. Your job is to change the system and help this girl who is on a downward spiral. I try to listen with my third ear; always searching for the isomorphic patterns and structural splits. This girl is not going to school. She's not doing what she needs to be doing in order to have a good future. She does whatever she wants. Is that true?

T: Um, I don't have reason to believe that it's not true.

HCF: Ok. if you look at the architecture of the system, there's not a good boundary between the generations if Mom is afraid to search her room. Is it against the law in Hawaii to smoke marijuana?

T: Yes, except for medicinal use.

Commentary: The isomorph is conflict avoidance and it creates a weak generational hierarchy. She's breaking the law, and the mom is not upset about it. The parents are both avoiding the conflicts; the mother will not go into her bedroom for fear of offending her, and the father is okay with poor grades, Ds. They are both failing their daughter. And yet, there is a financial plan for her to attend college.

With the isomorphs in mind, I suggest to my colleague to continue with the Intensity, support and challenge the parents to pull together, and create a hierarchy. Give this lost girl some direction and, if necessary, consequences.

Case Five: Electively Mute

B: This is the case we discussed previously. A selectively mute girl who does not speak at home or out of the house. The family accommodates to her. Her sister has even learned sign language so that she can function better as her megaphone. I remember that my strategy was to try and cut down the ways in which the family would accommodate and help her out, which I believe is maintaining her mutism. There was a team member who was new to the service, I think it was her first day, and she said, "That's awful, you're going to cause the girl to be distressed." And I replied, "Yes, that's going to be part of the therapy." Now my concern is that the parents and the sister of this girl are going to say, "You're going to cause our daughter to get more depressed and more distressed if we do this."

And I just realized, the team has now taken on this over-protective stance. We have a 15-year-old who hasn't been to school for a year, and her trajectory is so bad.

Commentary: The split between the professionals is untenable. I suggest that you sit down with the team and come to an agreement on the data/measurement that would demonstrate progress for this young girl. For example, the number of words spoken in a period of time: a morning, a day, expanding to a week. You agree to support their interventions for two months as progress is tracked. If there is no change, then they will agree to support your interventions. Bateson's (1972) concepts of symmetrical and complementary sequences are relevant. The present interactional pattern between you and the team is symmetrical; competitive, like a tennis match. You are at loggerheads. You have one position and they have one that is directly opposite. I am suggesting a new pattern—a counter-isomorph, complementary, a collaboration. If you and the team agree on the two-month trial, it represents a new, corrective isomorphic pattern.

Right now, there is no pressure on her to change. A gentle, systemic reorganization, such that the family does less for her and she does more for herself, is what you might suggest.

Case Six: Grand Rounds Case

I was visiting a community hospital in the United States and participated in their case discussion.

Dr. S: The parents described her past history: she always had attachment issues, it was very difficult to get her to stay in day-care. Mom told a story about when she was in primary school and didn't want to go; she would drop her off and turn to walk to the car. As she lifted the handle on the car door, she was surprised to find the youngster was directly behind her. She did eventually settle in primary school. They had been living overseas and when they returned home she was put in a class that her parents felt was too high for her; she struggled for a while but eventually she seemed to catch up. She's never read a book. She likes her devices, and she spends lots of time on those. When they take her devices away, she is inconsolable. She will not respond to them until she's given her device back.

The parents weren't happy for her to take medication; the child wasn't either. I was suggesting to them that she was very obviously depressed, she had anxiety and panic, and what she also revealed was that she had intrusive thoughts that had gone on for years. She described them: she would be talking to someone, and she would be thinking about choking them. She has great difficulty getting her thoughts to go away. She did have a ritual around food, but no others. She has one close friend and doesn't have any others; she only wants the one. She appeared obsessional, somewhat a loner, doesn't get along with her sisters. Mom is a psychologist. In any case, they didn't want any medication, they thought something to help her sleep and they'd like something natural, etc. We tried some sleep meds but they didn't work. They did agree on paroxetine. Then over the next number of days, she attended to another therapist when I was away. She was now saying overtly that she was hearing voices, she was seeing strange people, and she could hear them talking to her. The doctor suggested a low dose of quetiapine, 50 mg, and the parents agreed. She complained of side effects and the parents immediately stopped it.

We eventually negotiated, she would restart the quetiapine. She's continued throughout with the paroxetine. I saw her yesterday, and her parents are saying that she has considerably improved. Dad felt that she has improved since starting the quetiapine. Mom was saying, "No, it's not the quetiapine, she was beginning to improve anyway, and I think it's the paroxetine and her mood is getting better." I don't know, to be honest, what is happening, but that's where we are with her at the moment. I wondered about whether there was something organic. Seeing her yesterday, it didn't feel organic; there was nothing there suggesting that. Any ideas?

HCF: Dr. S, one question, is she going to school?

Dr. S: She's not going to school. Since the beginning, the parents date the problems back six months ago. They say that prior to this she was her normal self. There were some incidents at school, and she said she had a meltdown because her best friend was moved to another group. She said she felt acutely embarrassed. I don't know what else will have gone on at school. I think she is somebody who could very easily have been bullied at school. This year they negotiated that she would go two days a week, until fairly recently; she stopped going altogether.

HCF: *So, she now has school avoidance in addition to the other problems.*

Dr. S: Yes, she's certainly avoiding school now. There was another incident where she had a meltdown while out shopping for a dress with her dad. Mom works, they both work, but dad works mostly from home and does most of the childcare. She had a meltdown when she couldn't find a dress that suited her.

Dr. N: I was just going to ask, in terms of organicity, is she fully oriented? How about her cognition?

Dr. S: Yes, it seems there is no impairment of consciousness, she seems oriented in time, place, and person, yeah. There's nothing that feels organic about it. The other oddity is that among the hallucinations she described are olfactory hallucinations, which we don't certainly see very often. She smells cookies baking when there's no such stimulus about. But apart from that, there's nothing suggesting organicity when I see her.

Dr. L: And have those symptoms resolved with the quetiapine and paroxetine, the olfactory hallucinations? Have they gone away?

Dr. S: I don't know, to be honest with you. Yesterday, when I saw her, she didn't want to answer any direct questions, so I don't know if they've gone away or not. The parents thought that she seemed to be less distressed about things, but nobody's clear whether the hallucinations have actually gone. I didn't pursue them because she didn't want it pursued. It seemed to me that their presence had appeared fairly suddenly. I'd seen mom asking her about them in a manner that I felt was leading. "Are you hearing the voices now?" I've been reluctant; did not want to reinforce the notion.

Dr L: I imagine that Dr. L was asking because if they don't improve, alongside the other symptoms, with the antipsychotics, that might be an indication to pursue some investigations with an EEG, etc.

Dr. S: Indeed.

HCF: *Were there any changes in the family at the point at which the problem emerged?*

Dr. S: No, not any changes that I'm aware of at this point. Our psychologist who visited noted that there did seem to be conflict between mom and dad which I've not seen. When describing things, they correct one another quite a bit. The psychologist felt it was more than that, that they were sitting, arms folded, opposite the couch, glaring at one another; but I didn't see that. Again, they seem suspicious of too much questioning. Not suspicious, exactly; but they want the focus to be on the child, on her pathology and symptoms. I'm going gingerly with what's happening with the family. There's nothing obvious in the family, apart from their kind of correcting one another. It's really not fair to draw implications from that because they're under a lot of stress with this girl because she is quite dramatic in her acting out, and it would be surprising if they weren't going to get on each other's nerves around some of the time.

Dr. L: But the olfactory hallucinations are quite unusual. I think the only time I've seen this in depression is when I've seen kids with psychotic depression. And so, they're probably the only bit where I would be going, "Ooh, it's organic," and perhaps wondering about, you know, getting a bit of a work-up, a scan, and an EEG or something like that.

Dr. S: Indeed. I did talk to them about the possibility of a hospital admission with a view to seeing her away from the family, but she's opposed to the hospital, and they are as well.

Dr. L: Did you say you diagnosed her with psychotic depression? I think smelling cookies and cupcakes is unusual. With adults, they smell horrible things; like thinking their body smells, or they have cancer and can smell themselves rotting.

Dr. S: Yeah, there was nothing depressive in that. I'm not sure about the olfactory hallucinations. As I say, it did prick my ears up as something unusual and a bit worrying, but it's going along with auditory and visual hallucinations which are coordinated. You know, it was almost always factitious when they appeared.

Dr. N: Has she been reading about psychosis?

Dr. S: She may well have been, I don't know, she spends her life on the phone, on the internet, either playing games or searching around YouTube, but I don't know how much she's been reading. Certainly, she's had me questioning her about those symptoms. She's had others, and she's got mom, and kind of all of us focused on these psychotic symptoms so I think we may all have helped to blossom the thing.

Dr. N: Do you get the sense talking with her that they may be fabricated or factitious?

Dr. S: I don't get a sense of that from her. I mean, she's very reluctant to describe them, she describes them better to the case manager. She did suggest that some of her behaviors might be for secondary gain. The thing that makes me feel it's possibly factitious is this thing of the coordinating hallucinations, and the drama of everything. So, I'm not sure where I go next. When I discussed with them yesterday, I said, "Well, we'll certainly continue with the paroxetine but I don't want to continue with the quetiapine for too long."

Dr. N: Yeah.

Dr. S: I'm hoping that this psychotic side resolves fairly quickly and I don't have to make difficult decisions about antipsychotics. The parents are also opposed to her taking antipsychotics.

HCF: You might broaden the lens and assess this girl's context. You could have a family therapist work with the family and address the issues the psychologist noted. If the family's unstable, having a daughter who's manifesting psychiatric symptomatology would defuse their conflict and stabilize them.

Dr. S: Indeed. If that were the purpose, it is succeeding. They are doing round-the-clock minding of her, with dad sleeping in the hallway outside her room at night. Yeah, they are certainly working together on this matter.

HCF: Right. Not exactly together, if he is in the hallway and out of the couple's bed. The daughter becomes the de facto bundling board; keeping her parents apart.

Dr. S: I don't know whether she has to be dramatic and present all these kinds of symptoms in order just to express ordinary distress.

HCF: Right. Well, the more dramatic, the more attention it gets from the parents, and the more it deters the conflict.

Dr. S: Indeed, indeed, yeah.

HCF: Shopping with her father does suggest distance from the mother. Is the mother not available?

Dr. S: Mother works. On one occasion when the case manager wanted to see the child with mom at home, mom said she was far too busy, she had seven cases that day and she just didn't have time. So, but again, you know, we're taking snapshots and drawing conclusions from that, but it does appear mom is busy and working outside the home. The husband/father does something complicated with computers and marketing, which he's able to do from home.

Dr L.: Well, I also think being a mental health professional and having significant mental health problems in your child is a very vulnerable place to be, isn't it?

Dr. S: Indeed, indeed.

Dr. N: Was this helpful, S?

Dr. S: Yeah, it's helpful to stand back from it and hear that there's nothing too obvious sticking out. But, yeah, I'm feeling kind of overwhelmed with piles of information all coming in dribs and drabs, and a clearly very distressed little girl.

Dr. L: Would you do an MRI brain scan? A young person with possible psychosis, just to make sure you don't miss anything?

Dr. S: Yeah, I mean that was one of the things that I was hoping smarter people than myself might have an opinion on.

Dr. N: I'm not sure that I'm smarter than you, but when I was working in the early psychosis team, I just always thought that if you're young enough to present with a psychosis you deserve a brain scan, you know.

Dr. N: Neurologists are always really helpful at the Children's Hospital, and they've got a low threshold with symptoms that are a bit unusual for zipping through a brain scan; and a good neurological examination. If they're really concerned they'll do an LP and look for antibodies. And the good thing is she's 13 so they'll see her. You know, once she hits 15, it's a lot harder with the adult neurologists.

Dr. S: Right, ok.

Dr. L: Yeah, I think you could make a reasonable argument for early psychotic symptoms. And as far as scanning a new psychosis, most of us would prefer that a brain was scanned. I mean, the yield is ridiculously low, but if it was my kid I'd want that to happen.

Dr. S: We don't routinely scan people here or ask for scans, and the other thing is that we don't routinely check for encephalitis and such.

Dr. L: There's a movement in early intervention suggesting that stuff should be done. Certainly, you know, a lot of places would see that as just routine...

Dr. N: It's 7%, I think, in people who've got no organic signs whatsoever, with early psychosis.

Commentary: The treatment team is stuck. They appear to be going around in circles. A singular focus on early psychosis with the added suspicion of factitious symptomatology calls for a very broad lens. The family context needs full assessment, especially the suspicion of the conflictual parental dyad that was observed by the psychologist. Based on this snapshot, the only isomorph identified is that of a rigid treating system. There were major glaring bits of suspicious data: the psychologist's report and the girl's difficulties at school that might lead to factitious illness. Consulting to this professional system, I would challenge the isomorph of their rigidity, their blind spot for context, and encourage them to work with the family and the school to assess if the dynamics were commensurate with this presentation.

Case Seven: Internet Gaming Disorder

B: At the child and adolescent mental health service where I work, I said, "I'm sorry, I'm not quite sure what we're doing here." Mom was requesting that someone from the mental health service go up to see her son and find some way of putting him into detention to treat him. The clinician who took the phone call agreed. I think the whole system kind of agreed, concurred with mom, that that's what was needed. It got to the point where they lined up to find another clinician from another service who had expertise in treating internet gaming disorder, whatever that is. To come in and provide an intervention for the young person.

The interesting thing about this case, from my perspective, is that one parent is assisting all the clinicians who are involved in making decisions about the treatment of this kid. I had the advantage, I guess, where I had not met the kid, not seen the mom; I was not drawn into it. I asked a couple of questions, "Has mom ever been to a session with anybody else? Has there been a parent intervention? Any attempts at a system-based intervention?"

The answer was no; nothing really at all, not even a school counselor. I suggested that maybe mom would like to come in for a session; mom and grandma, that's where we should start.

What happened? The other members of the team felt that was a bad idea. The questions that got thrown at me were the questions that mom had asked in the emergency department, "Could he be depressed? We need to know what's going on with him; he deserves to be treated." Then they said, "mom's too scared, she can't do anything, and all of that." One parent resembled or represented the mental health service; another parent, I thought of as "the mom." I kind of held my ground for a while.

I ended up in a bit of a battle. What I realized, after listening to H, is that I didn't try an Intensity argument. We ended up in a battle where nobody talked about what the outcome might be for the child and all I talked about was the evidence base and the importance of the system of working with the parents and that hadn't been done. I didn't do the thing where I would say, "if your child does not go to school he will deteriorate, and yes, he will become very depressed, and so we have to do the thing that we know is best." I think that would have been a useful intervention at the time. I'll leave it there because those are my thoughts.

HCF: *They call this an "internet disorder"?*

B: People love calling it "internet gaming disorder." I don't subscribe to the construct...

HCF: *It's the medicalization of the behavior.*

B: Yeah.

HCF: What isn't normal is the school avoidance; it is a grave concern and must be treated.

B: Look, it's interesting. Over the past few years I've seen a lot of this. Prolonged school refusal or school non-attendance, parents not in a power situation, or not at the top of the hierarchy, for a variety of reasons. Often it's single parents. What it gets labeled as is a child problem, rather than anybody thinking about parental system issues. Maybe they think about it but it is just too hard.

Commentary: There are two issues: the mom wants the system to control her child, and the treatment team lacks consensus—they are not in agreement. There is a Batesonian symmetrical struggle between the consultant and the community team that is treating the young person. Mom's search for specialists for this "disease" serves as a deflection from the real issue, the parental disempowerment. I suspect that the parents (mom and grandmother) do not agree and they are triangulating the boy.

Mom, in her quest for a pill to fix the "disease," avoids the confrontation. There are so many isomorphs but I suggest that you select the most immediate, the discordant clinical team. Following from the Elective Mute Case, I would attempt to transform the treating system to one of the complementary sequences. I would, almost simultaneously, work with the mother and grandmother; do your best to Join with them, so they can begin to establish the required hierarchy. Get him to school and control the internet; they do pay for the Wi-Fi.

Case Eight: Polyfest Case

HCF: Listen for the underlying structure of the family; that is what you're changing.

B: I tend to look for complexities, and I find it difficult to hold the fact that something so simple could be so useful. A reflection, not a question.

HCF: There is an unlearning; I felt exactly the same way when I started. So, let's try this, a bit of an experiment. H, why don't you tell us more about your case?

H: My case from last time? The enmeshment between adopted son and the mother, and somewhat placid father, I guess. We had a session the week after we all last met, which de-railed almost immediately, with the son barging into the room and making a request to go to a festival we have here, it's called Polyfest. It's kind of like the biggest cultural gathering for Pacific Islanders in NZ.

However, the way that he approached the situation was with a lot of sass. The parents started asking him pretty reasonable questions: Who will you be going with? What time will you be back? And he spat some venom back at them, basically saying, "I'm 17 years old, I should be able to do what I want, I don't have to tell you anything about what I'm doing," and this pattern just continued to escalate. I said, "Look, can we stop? M, can you just go out of the room, hang out with your youth worker for a little bit; I need to speak to your parents about something." Then I asked, "How long are you guys willing to play this role in M's life, where you have no power; you don't make any decisions, and you just go round and round the carousel with him, asking him questions? I think you two should decide whether or not you think this behavior is something you should tolerate or not, and decide that together. I'm going to go outside and I'll talk to M for five to ten minutes, and then when we come back, hopefully you guys can come up with some sort of decision about what you want to do here." I left the room and spoke with M for a while; he was very upset, his parents "treat him like a baby" and this sort of thing, so I just sort of sat there and listened to him. But really what I was doing was giving the parents some time to create this decision. I think for weeks and weeks I've been trying to encourage them to utilize some sort of consequence or initiate some sort of boundary with him about how he speaks to them, and the amount of pressure that he puts on them. I think what he is really calling for is, "Give me some boundaries, give me a clear lane of operation," I suppose. When we went into the room again, M and I sat down, and I said, "Ok, do you have anything you want to say about M's behavior?" And they said, "Well, we really don't like the way that you ask us things, you know it's not what you're saying that's the problem, it's how you're saying it, so we've decided you can't go to this festival, and we'll be cutting off your internet access through your phone for the week." He would no longer be able to coordinate with his friends, and so forth. I thought, "Hallelujah, they're finally on the same page about something, they've made a decision, and they have put their foot down despite their fear of his reactions." Of course he exploded out of his chair, "I hate you guys, it's lucky I don't f*** you up," and all this sort of thing, so he got threatening. I just looked at them and cued them not to react, and they didn't, and he stormed out of the room. Following that, I sat with the parents for a little while, and M refused to re-engage in the session and went home. "Now, the really really important thing for you guys is to make sure that you don't fold back on yourselves and succumb to any pressure that he tries to put on you, from now on." And lo and behold, before I was even finished talking to them, M rang his mother and started basically abusing her over the phone, "If I ever see you again, I'm going to beat you up, I can't believe you've done this to me, I can't live without Instagram," so, bargaining through threats; bargaining and threatening at the same time, it was very intense. "You know, I told you you could expect this, it's now your decision whether you want to carry this new pattern, I suppose, forward to the time that you said you would. It's very important that you hold on to your follow-through, otherwise he will exploit the cracks in your parenting again." That went ok for about three days, and then over the course of the weekend he managed to call his parents enough and be enough of a good boy to get access to his Instagram account. His parents control the account, and of course coordinate his movements and he went to the Polyfest.

B: Remind me how old he is again?

H: He's 17 years old.

B: Ok.

H: As far as I was concerned, I think that him having exposure to social environments is probably a good thing for him, however, I think he needs a lot more work with what's going on with the background of his life before he starts launching himself into the foreground. I think he would have been fine to go to that Polyfest, either on his own or with his friends, with the support of staff, but I was of a position where I would much rather he go with the support and permission of his parents, so his parents would bail him out if he got into any trouble that day. He kind of shot himself in the foot straight away, when approaching the problem.

HCF: H, let me ask you this, he's a resident in your program?

H: Yes.

HCF: He's living with you guys?

H: Yep.

HCF: Do you think this intervention was successful or unsuccessful?

H: Well, if I'm looking at the outcome I would say unsuccessful, because he disobeyed his parents' wishes and got what he was going to do anyway.

HCF: How did he disobey his parents' wishes?

H: I suppose, getting access to Instagram again...

HCF: But his parents gave him permission.

H: Yeah, yeah, that's right, so I think it's more of a failure on them sticking to their goal than him and his behavior.

HCF: So what do other people think?

B: Because I have only one session with people, I look at the end of your session and I think it was a success; certainly three days later it was no longer a success but you had three days of success. If I had known the family I would have been walking out pleased.

HCF: Anybody else?

S: That was my thought too, because the parents did exactly what you wanted them to do. When you left the room they worked together and came up with a plan together and that was the Enactment. And like B said, you know, maybe the success only lasted three days but it sounds like that's three more days than they had had in the past.

N: Yeah, and I'm curious, H, did the parents agree together to give him permission to access his Instagram? Is that something they came to together?

H: That's actually bang on the head about what I was going to say from this last Thursday. That was the question that I asked them, "So, who decided to put Instagram back on," and of course it was mom who folded first, and dad sort of just went along with his wife, and that's his typical pattern.

Commentary: The parents were together in presenting the consequence while in the session. Some days later, the mother capitulated. This is a manifestation of the split between the parents, the evidence of triangulation, which is the etiology of his misbehavior, suggesting more work is necessary. Remember, our role is to change the isomorph. While it may be good for him to have the experience of going to Polyfest, our job is looking from 35,000 feet at the destructive pattern and changing it.

Case Nine: Wild Child Referral

I consulted by Zoom to an agency in the United States regarding this out-of-control boy. The staff was concerned that this boy was losing his childhood by his long periods of incarceration.

Tony is a 17-year-old boy who is so dangerous to the community he has been locked up 15 times, for a total of 800 days. Each time he is released, he quickly steals a car; there are 14 cases of stolen cars on the police books implicating Tony. These often result in high-speed chases, always driving on the wrong side of the road. His biological father is deceased. His mother has a history of being deeply traumatized by the police when she was young. She is addicted to methylphenidate, deals drugs, and is heavily involved with gangs. She worked in the past as a prostitute. She and her present partner have violent episodes that require police intervention. There are five boys in this family ranging in age from 21 to ten. The grandparents are deceased and there are no aunts or uncles who have been identified. Tony's 21-year-old brother, the oldest sibling, has just been released from jail. All the boys come home to the mother, but it does not last. She or her boyfriend kicks them out.

Tony was diagnosed with fetal alcohol syndrome (FAS) when young. His ability to read and write and calculate has not been reported. When in lockup, he does write rap music to pass the time. There are currently 35 charges pending, including burglary and car theft, and he is due in court. When he leaves lockup he is placed in non-profit residential agencies; he usually elopes within two days.

When attending the Zoom meeting to discuss a pending court case for Tony, the police, his lawyer, and a social worker agreed to disagree. Tony, sitting alongside his older and younger brothers, who were there for support, told his lawyer he wanted to stay in the community. The social worker asked Tony to choose a mandated residential program where he would like to be committed for his community incarceration. The police wanted the judge to lock him up in prison. The decision of the judge is pending.

Commentary: The relationship between social service and the teenager is surprisingly enmeshed. All these years, every time he was released from lock up, he would be sent to a community residential program and elope within two days. He would proceed to maraud the community. Fifteen charges resulted from this last elopement. The social workers feel so badly for him, with his repeated lockups, that they advocate for him to return to residential care in the community; this has never been successful, doing the same thing and expecting different results.

The disengaged family offers no supervision, no housing, and the parental hierarchy is absent. The brothers offer no parental substitution, with the older ones in and out of prison. The overall isomorph is chaos. The professionals disagree, the siblings are disempowered and in trouble, and the mother and her partner are in a violent relationship. The police and the social service agency are locked in a symmetrical hold. They disagree and cannot accommodate to reach consensus. The diagnosis of FAS serves to lower the expectations of the lad and engenders sympathy and forgiveness from the professionals. The consequences from the legal and social service system do not bother this youngster—they "roll off his back." He enjoys lockup and quickly finds a way to return. His true freedom is the residential community setting—a pass-through solution.

One positive note, as I mentioned, all the boys come back to the mother. The team has decided to capitalize on this aspect and provide ongoing support to the mother to help her parent her sons, developing a functional parenting hierarchy.

Summary

One of the great powers in family therapy is perceiving and transforming isomorphic patterns. From this generic meta perspective, the clinician focuses on the deep structures of the family system, leading to better outcomes. On Sunday afternoons, I am always urging these clinicians to get contemporary; look at the patterns in front of you and avoid distractions.

10

OUR CHALLENGE

This book is filled with good news. RBA, new to our field, has great promise for mental health clinics, private practitioners, programs large and small, and populations. Similarly, IST, an effective family therapy, has proven results. But there are still dire problems. The research findings that psychotherapy and psychopharmacology are not effective have sounded the alarm by Leichsenring and Ioannidis.

A few years ago, Dr. Tom Insel left his directorship of The National Institute of Mental Health (NIMH), considered a cathedral of the world's leading research institutes in biological psychiatry, for Google's health division.

I spent 13 years really pushing on the neuroscience and genetics of mental disorders, and when I look back on that, I realize that while I think I succeeded at getting lots of really cool papers published by cool scientists at fairly large costs—I think $20 billion— I don't think we moved the needle in reducing suicide, reducing

DOI: 10.4324/9781003161257-11

hospitalizations, improving recovery for the tens of millions of people who have mental illness. I hold myself accountable for that.

(Rogers, 2017)

The evidence-based medicine movement—sometimes limiting creativity—may have been one of the major barriers to his success. Lisbeth B. Schorr, a Harvard lecturer and Senior Fellow at the Center for Study of Social Policy (CSSP), together with her colleague, Frank Farrow, formed a group in 2011 called "Friends of Evidence." They were researchers, practitioners, and thought leaders who shared the conviction that new ways of working required changes in the types of evidence gathered and how to use that evidence. In one of the symposia that they convened, the paper "Expanding the Evidence Universe: Doing Better by Knowing More" (Schorr & Farrow, 2011) was presented in the spirit of furthering discussion, prompting additional debate and contributing to the shared urgency for moving forward. They said that innovative, purposeful, and evidence-informed strategies could improve life outcomes for children, strengthen families, and build healthy, safe, and supportive communities (Schorr & Farrow, 2011).

The group discussed that research and experience over the past two decades have provided more knowledge than ever before about what it takes to improve outcomes for disadvantaged children and families. But that knowledge has not been successful in achieving better outcomes in the magnitude that matches the need. They believed that the failure to marshal the full extent of available knowledge, apply it to complex problems, and generate new knowledge from the efforts, was missing. They stated that the definition of what counts as credible evidence must expand. There should be agreement that the value of many kinds of interventions can be assessed, weighed, understood, and acted upon without having to be proven through experimental methods (Schorr & Farrow, 2011).

I wonder if these compelling points of view have shifted the tide away from the narrow focus on experimental evidence of program impact as postulated by Lisbeth Schorr in the Stanford Social Innovation Review in 2016 (Schorr, 2016).

The following anecdote represents the sentiments held by many clinicians, especially family therapists. A colleague of mine from the Midwest sought my advice regarding an innovative youth program she hoped to establish for adolescent offenders in the local penal system. She was locked out of funding and referrals. Why? The government agency, funding these initiatives, mandated that they use only evidence-based treatment programs. "This mandate makes me very sad; we have an excellent program that is not available to the very youth who have the most desperate need," she complained. "The rigidity of the agency stifled my creative program," she remarked. In my experience, I cautiously suggested to her, this was not uncommon for clinicians. The managers do have a valid position—how can they ensure the probability that there will be good outcomes for their constituents, especially when they're spending public money? To counter this conundrum, I recommended to my colleague that she become more knowledgeable about RBA and the Turning the Curve tool. With this, she could track her own data and document her existing program's effectiveness. Then, with this alternative method of "real-world" evidence, approach the gatekeepers.

Lisbeth Schorr says the paucity of good measurement tools can be a formidable barrier to maintaining accountability, managing by results, continuously improving quality, and assessing impact in complex initiatives (Schorr & Farrow, 2011). Strengthen measurement for accountability and learning by: developing appropriate measures for smaller geographic units; developing metrics to capture all critical work; creating appropriate interim measures; and helping all stakeholders to emphasize and work with shared results (Schorr & Farrow, 2011). In the RBA tradition of measuring, the Turning the Curve tool is an excellent measurement tool that could be easily adapted for Midwest adolescent offenders. The barrier for my colleague may be removed.

Thomas Schwandt, an evaluation guru, said in the book *What Counts as Credible Evidence in Applied Research and Evaluation Practice?* (cited in Schorr 2016) that the term "evidence-based" must be interpreted with caution: "To claim that evidence may figure importantly in our decisions is one thing; to claim it is foundational for our actions is another. We would well be advised to talk about evidence-informed decision making instead" (Schorr, 2016).

Mark Friedman counters that the "evidence-only policy" actively discourages partnerships and community involvement. If the government only funds research-proven practices, then those who can participate in these types of discussions are effectively limited to the academic community. This approach alienates the community and lessens the clinician's opportunity for success, simply by failing to utilize community problem-solving tactics (Friedman, 2015).

> The research world can only tell us a fraction of what we need to know. Thus, we must make sure that we use our common sense, our life experiences, and our knowledge of the communities within which we live. ... there must be room ... for innovation.
>
> (Friedman 2015)

Vincent DeVita, MD, in his book, *The Death of Cancer*, wrote that evidence-based guidelines for the treatment of cancer are "backward looking." He wrote, "With cancer, things change too rapidly for doctors to be able to rely on yesterday's guidelines for long. Reliance on such standards inhibits doctors from trying something new" (Schorr, 2016).

Don Berwick, a health policy reformer, and a colleague in the Friends of Evidence Project, described the situation and offered a way to get better results in this complex world (Schorr 2016). He said that we must draw on, generate, and apply a broader range of evidence to take account of all factors that we have largely neglected in the past. Build the political will by becoming smarter in how we approach the generation, analysis, and application of knowledge and evidence (Berwick, 2007).

The "Friends" project, to expand the definition of acceptable data, offered a new beginning of inclusivity in mental health. All those clinicians who are contributing important and innovative outcomes finally have a ticket into the club of evidence. I am reminded, however, of a fable from Ancient Greece, where a man is looking at the stars and falls into a well. For those of us on the front line, the ground beneath us has many hazards.

A few years ago, I accepted a locum position for ten days in a child and adolescent psychiatric outpatient clinic in another New Zealand community. I traveled the night before and arrived at the clinic at 8:00 am as instructed. Entering the building was the first hurdle. No one answered the bell; I could not reach anyone by phone to guide my way into the facility. It was the first hint of the dysfunctional system I was soon to encounter.

A staff member happened by, and I gained entry on his swipe card. Once inside, I was summarily told that my first patient was scheduled for 9 am, and when I finally located an office, I discovered that there was not a computerized patient record. There was no orientation process, just the stack of paper files for the patients scheduled for the day.

As the day progressed, I noted that each professional simply "stayed in their lane." They were friendly and appeared to be committed professionals; they were definitely tired. I was struck by the absence of measuring patient progress; there were no tools available and they were still using pen and paper. There was no organized system of care; it felt like "parallel play." Examining the files, one was aware that the problems did not resolve, what was constant was a continuous retinue of puzzled clinicians. There was no consensus on the desired outcomes for the cases. I longed for an RBA-based, family therapy-oriented clinic—an organized system where everyone was focused on common outcomes.

During my 10-day tenure, I consulted with a variety of distressed families. I quickly realized my role was to provide medication consultations, mostly Ritalin. Of course, many, if not all, of these young people were misdiagnosed with ADHD; a narrow diagnostic attempt to fix the child. It did not take me long, however, to notice the lack of cohesiveness. The clinical staff (i.e., clinicians/therapists, social workers, nurses) were not functioning as a treatment team; there was no active collaboration to provide the best treatment for clients/patients. They did not encourage the family to become active participants in the treatment process. Most importantly, there were no commonly agreed-upon goals.

Not only was RBA missing but so was IST. Diagnostically, there were no attempts to seek understanding of the children and family contexts maintaining the presenting symptomatology. The children appeared to be growing up all alone in the woods.

Among my many consultations, I have chosen only three patients to indicate the dizzying myopia. There were sadly so many more.

Case One: Bonnie

Bonnie, a nine-year-old girl, presented with anxiety. She complained, "I'm afraid of the wind." She was afraid to venture outside the confines of her home. Her mother, Beth, complained that Bonnie's symptoms were not only profoundly upsetting to the family, but, most importantly, they severely restricted Bonnie's activities. When I met with this lovely, young girl, I was impressed. Bonnie was expressive, outgoing, and friendly.

Beth shared with me that "the problem" began three years ago. And, I asked, "What changed at that time—in the family and or in Bonnie's life?" You probably guessed Beth's answer, "Well, nothing much happened, except my husband and I separated." I asked, "Okay, so how's that going?" Beth reported that her ex-husband, Jim, was now dating someone new and that she had "friction" with this new girlfriend, Jessica. Jessica constantly called her "the Bio-Mom" in front of Bonnie, which upset her. And there was a preponderance of drama during Bonnie's visitations with Jim and Jessica.

Bonnie was distressed, and her parents, Beth and Jim, as well as Jessica, didn't help her. More specifically, Beth and Jim triangulated their young daughter. It appeared that Jessica may also be the homeostatic maintainer, as Beth described their attempts at making peace between the two households. It was no wonder that Bonnie was suffering from anxiety, given the rancor and dysfunction in the parental subsystem. The family (the two-house parental system) was not functioning well, and that contributed to Bonnie's stress. There was no fixed visitation schedule, even after three years. Upcoming visitations would occur at the last minute.

As I was reading Bonnie's medical records, I was shocked at the limited services this girl had received. In fact, there was only individual therapy with a psychologist, who was solely focused on whether she had ADHD or major cognitive problems. She had had numerous psychiatric assessments to no avail.

Additionally, the father had recently been discharged from a psychiatric hospital. It did not appear that there was any consideration of the amount of stress that all the family members had been suffering. There were also no contextual formulations in regard to her "fear of the wind." With this symptom, Bonnie could not easily leave her home and go to her dad and Jessica's house. Bonnie's clinical team requested a consultation so she could be placed into a diagnostic category and offered medication (which I did not do). Did they really think adding Ritalin would stop this girl's poetic fear of the wind?

I began the process of de-triangulating this young girl and made recommendations that she be seen by the family therapist ASAP to work
with all family members to address the contextual issues.

Case Two: Jimmy

Jimmy, a ten-year-old boy, had been referred because a previous psychologist diagnosed him with ADHD. They were seeking a prescription
for Ritalin. I consulted with Jimmy and his family. His mother, Sally, was
extremely distraught. Apparently, the day before, the teacher had called
to say that Jimmy had written on a chalkboard, "Jimmy is dead." He had
also drawn a picture of a stick figure raising his hands in the air. Jimmy
presented as a shy, reticent boy, cooperative and thoughtful. He told me
that he was bullied by his sister, Belle, who was four years older, and he
was afraid of her. The psychologist and the mother strongly held that
Jimmy needed psychotropic medication. But, his father, Matthew, who
had been diagnosed early in his life with ADHD, had very strong feelings
against psychostimulants. Matthew feared that the medications would
effectively "squash" his son's creativity.

Seeing the parents alone, with Jimmy in the reception area, I shared
my opinion that "Jimmy is caught between the two of you. In that regard,
he can never be comfortable. He will always disappoint one of you." The
father was blocking the psychostimulant on an emotional basis, disre-
garding the psychologist's diagnosis and recommendation. This position, while triangulating, also kept the system "stuck." I explained that,
"Jimmy is in the middle of your marriage, and, as a result, he and the
whole family are being affected."

After speaking with Matthew and Sally, it became increasingly clear
that the current family system was not only rife with triangulation but
also rigid. I have learned through my many years of practice that suicidal
ideation (i.e., suicidal thoughts, attempts, and actions) often occurs when
the threshold for change is so high in individuals (i.e., family members)
that they manifest a symptom, like suicidal ideation, to try to effectively
jar the system.

Meeting with Jimmy, alone, he made it clear that he too was not in
favor of Ritalin. He also stated that his previous counselor instructed

him to stop telling people he was suicidal——yes, you read that correctly! When I asked Jimmy why, he explained that the counselor told him when he tells others he wants to kill himself, it upsets them. I thought that Jimmy's counselor had applied a muzzle and that was dangerous. Jimmy needed to be free to express his feelings, especially suicidal ideation, to those people who could help him. The counselor, like the father, similarly assumed the position of homeostatic maintainer when he embargoed Jimmy from mentioning his suicidality.

This well-meaning, struggling family needed good professional help. Sally and Matthew needed to agree on the Ritalin question, so Jimmy would not feel he was betraying one parent or the other. I also recommended that Matthew and Sally quickly intervene with the bullying committed by his sister. I did not prescribe the medication and instead asked them to take time to think it over and get back to the clinic. I warned the manager of the clinic that Jimmy's counselor may be contributing unwarranted risk for suicidality.

Case Three: Allan

Allan, a 16-year-old boy, lived with his grandmother, Mattie, and two aunts, Gloria and Ruth. Allan had been previously diagnosed with an intellectual disability and ulcerative colitis. Allan came to the clinic because Mattie had noticed an escalating level of anger and anxiety in him. She wanted to know if there were any psychotropic medications that could help him control these behaviors. Allan's biological mother, Elizabeth, suffered from repeated drug and alcohol problems and was not currently in his life. His biological father's location was unknown. During the consultation, I learned that Allan was in school and that he had a support worker to help him with his classes.

Allan presented as an easy-going, friendly young man, who was completely committed to his grandmother, Mattie, a sentiment that was manifestly reciprocated. When Allan was asked about his anxiety and anger, he was hesitant. In discussions with Mattie, she told me there was conflict with her daughters, who were her landlords. In addition, Allan said that he was unhappy with his support worker and increasingly they did not get along. Once again, I was presented with a "family system" that had multiple structural splits: Mattie with her adult daughters, and Allan with his minder.

Developmentally, Allan was in a difficult position. He was living in a context surrounded by people taking care of him; treating him as a "special child" and thereby keeping him from the important stretch and growth period of late adolescence. He loved to sail, and apparently, he was excellent at it, but his minder discounted this area of expertise. In this system, the prevailing isomorph was conflict avoidance, and this was very probably a sign of a psychosomatic family.

There was also Allan's chronic illness—ulcerative colitis (UC). I determined that what Allan needed most was an intervention to decrease the stressful relationships in his context. This ongoing stress may well have exacerbated his medical condition.

Easing Allan's anger and anxiety with medication would probably relieve some of his anxiety and placate the grandmother. If it was the only intervention, it would fail to address the painful relationship issues creating stress and anxiety.

They wanted a *deus ex machina*, a miracle to solve their relationship problems. I prescribed a mild anti-anxiety medication for the lad—along with my strong recommendation for family therapy to address their interpersonal issues and intervene with the minder who was contributing to Allan's dysphoria.

The treating professionals carelessly ignored these families and the opportunity to swiftly ameliorate their symptoms and transform the families to prevent future symptomatology. There's an old joke that typifies this failure. It's late in the night in a stadium, the football game ended hours earlier. In the empty parking lot, a policeman comes up to a man who is on all fours. He asks, "What exactly are you doing?" The man says, "Well, I've lost my keys and I'm searching for them." "Where did you lose them?" The searching man points to an area about 50 feet away. "Well, if you dropped them over there, why are you searching over here?" The man raises his head, points to a streetlight, and says, "The light's better here." In the same way, it is much more convenient in these clinics to work only with the individual. The problem, however, is the keys are not with the individual patient, they are in the family context maintaining the symptoms.

Was this clinic the "poster child" for mental health clinics worldwide? I hoped not, but experience was telling me otherwise. Don Berwick, in his keynote address, *Quality, Mercy and the Moral Determinants of Health*, presented at the Institute for Healthcare Improvement (IHI) National Forum in 2019, and the subsequent article "The Moral Determinants of Health" (Berwick, 2020), sounded the alarm for the predicament we are in. Berwick said, "except for a few clinical preventative services, most hospitals and physician offices are repair shops, trying to correct the damage of causes collectively denoted, social determinants of health." Beyond the necessity of bearing witness, the moral imperative for mental health clinics is to address contemporary pressures within the broad context of families; do not hang the 'repair' on the sacrificed young person.

Anyone reading this book to this point knows that my recommendations for effective outcomes in mental health clinics require sound infrastructures like the RBA framework. Berwick's old faithfuls of patient safety and continuous quality improvement, reducing costs, and uncovering waste in health care systems remain relevant and should not be overlooked (Berwick et al., 2003). However, I would expand Berwick's concept of patient-centered care to "family and community-centered" care; an inclusivity of all stakeholders involved in solving problems. In the three cases that I discussed, the families simply appeared to deliver their children much like "Uber eats" delivers our takeaway meals. At least the Uber corporation has a tracking system that is downloaded to your mobile phone and you can locate the movements of your pizza during its journey. The irony that technology and innovation have lifted the world's population into a new way of living and working, while paper medical records pretend to document and share the patient's medical information, will be found out.

The medical records of these three youngsters did not disclose any parental dynamics; the influence of the parents on the presenting problems was absent. Berwick's concern with morality strikes at the heart of the problem in "the girl afraid of the wind." The medical system conspired using the medical model by focusing on the individual—pinning the problem on the girl.

In each one of these families, the parents are comfortably in their corners. Where is the humanity or mercy for these children? "Do they love their child, more than they hate each other?" is an ethical question. At what point do they drop their clenched fist for the good of the child? This is the existential question that countless families must face: When does the love for their child prevail?

Being at this clinic felt unsafe. The secret covenant with the youngster, asking him to hide his suicidality, required urgent attention. While I did alert the director of the Clinic, the lack of transparency in all of their practice left me uneasy. Once again, a clinician staying in their lane and practicing as the sole agent suggested that this was the Wild West. There was no organized system; there was no ability to track outcomes and measure the clinician's performance against quality measures.

In the ten days that I worked there, I continuously longed for the RBA framework so that this important community mental health clinic could better serve its children and families. On the last day of my locum contract, a farewell lunch, in the New Zealand tradition, was scheduled for me. I was unable to attend this function because separately, back-to-back patients had been booked, prohibiting this opportunity to say goodbye to my colleagues. Near the end of the day, anxious to share my ideas for quality improvement, I invited myself into the office of the clinic manager. Within one minute, it was disappointingly obvious there was no interest in change. Too bad; I would have explained about the "nudge" concept and the need to include the family.

The highly influential book, Nudge, authored by Thaler and Sunstein in 2008, influenced governmental systems. The premise of the book is that a minor shift can create significant change. For many years, states could not get people to indicate on their driver licenses that they were willing to be organ donors, stranding many people without solutions to their grave medical problems. The "nudge" to the system was simple: check the box only if you do not want to donate; the assumption was that everyone was a donor unless they said no. Organ donations increased dramatically.

This simple nudge could be applied here to this clinic and other mental health clinics. Enroll the family as the client, not just the child. The enrolment form would require family members to be listed to fulfill enrolment. This opens the door widely for clinicians, and all stakeholders, to work with the parents, addressing family issues all requiring collaborating partners. This redefines the team's jurisdiction and responsibility.

Clinicians' loyalty to their professional guilds can interfere with collaboration. This danger is mitigated by a common focus on outcomes, where everyone together is held responsible. Of course, this requires fealty to tracking data. The disorganized mental health clinics, clinging to their status quo, prohibit innovation; they are treading water and unable to try something new and track effectiveness.

Today, everyone is tracking outcomes; even our eight-year-old granddaughter tracks her walking steps with a wristwatch. She reports weekly and monthly summaries. Recently, she completed a record-breaking day, walking 35,000 steps; she was thrilled. Now she is interested in goal setting and beating her personal best. Patients track their sleep cycles, hours of sleep, breathing patterns, and caloric intake, challenging the medical system to manage all of the generated data. Blockchain will likely be required. And yet, this mental health clinic is not measuring or tracking any outcomes; they could not answer the question, Is anybody better off?

All clinics should have a community resource specialist working with families on social and economic issues. To the extent that the family has more economic stability, there is less stress; everyone does better, especially the children. With economically disadvantaged families, it lessens the probability that their children will be removed, become conduct disordered, or spend time in the criminal justice system.

Silos of funding create roadblocks in treatments. They interfere with an organized system of care where integration of services can be required to reach the goals of treatment. This is the nemesis of those working in public systems. When the treatment team determines that the families need resources to facilitate their treatment goals, the required funds may not be there in "real time." Blended funding is considered the "holy grail" for those of us working in these public systems. Otherwise, each agency jealously guards its funds. If we're going to propose an ideal mental health clinic when working with families, pooled funding should be available.

The Field of Family Therapy

Transforming our beloved field of family therapy, we therapists must organize as one cohesive unit. As a field, we believe in systems, let's become one. Yes, of course, we love our treatment models, but, if we are going to do our part to rectify the poor worldwide outcomes, this will take all of us. It is sometimes unclear what family therapy model works best for specific problem areas.

This will require that client outcomes and program progress be tracked and published; we need to prove the effectiveness of our therapy. Those clinicians, the "local clinical scientists" at the coal face, who are tackling family problems, should be recognized for the monumental contribution they could make to the researched literature.

There is a mounting concern that treatment research, and the EBM model, are restricting valuable evidence and how to use that evidence. Lisbeth Schorr, in her paper, *Doing Better by Knowing More*, presented to the symposia that innovative, purposeful, and evidence-informed strategies could improve life outcomes for children. This is a challenge to the editors in our field (Schorr & Farrow, 2011).

I presented in these pages a simple, straightforward methodology to track performance. The key is to measure, measure, and measure some more! The Turning the Curve tool determines whether anybody is better off. The editors of our scientific journals need to follow Lisbeth Schorr's advice and expand the jurisdiction of acceptable data. We, from the coal face of families and communities, have much to contribute.

In closing, back to my Midwestern US roots, I am reminded of the license plates of Missouri, "The Show-Me State." This speaks to all clinicians. Become a local clinical scientist; show your evidence to the world that you are achieving good outcomes.

As the anthropologist Margaret Mead once said, "Never doubt that a small group of thoughtful, committed citizens can change the world—indeed, it's the only thing that ever has."

Let's change mental health care, our families need you.

APPENDIX

The inventory of IST/RBA Treatment Tools:

- IST Family Evaluation and Intervention Tools: IST Triangulation, Single Parent Scale, Homeostatic Maintainer Searchlight
- Treatment Algorithms: school avoidance, failing grades, conduct disorder, eating disorders
- Alphabet of Skills Worksheet: educating the family, search for strength, boundary making, joining, intensity, enactment, complementarity, unbalancing
- Windsor House Economic Opportunity Assessment and Intervention Tool
- Reflection Tool for Supervisees
- Consumer Feedback Evaluation Tool
- Clinician's Mastery Report
- IST/RBA Clinical Scorecard Worksheet
- Targeting Tool-Clinical Scorecard Worksheet

Re: Chapters 4, 5, and 8

IST Family Evaluation and Intervention

IST Triangulation Scale	Never (0)	Rarely (1)	Sometimes (2)	Often (3)	Always (4)
1. To what extent are the parents willing to sit in the room together?					
2. To what extent are the parents able to come to an agreement on a single point regarding their child?					
3. To what extent do the parents support one another in their expectations for their child's behavior?					
4. To what extent do the parents actively triangulate their child?					
5. To what extent do the parents recruit others into their conflict?					
6. To what extent are the parents able to agree on a specific consequence and confront their adolescent?					
Total score:					

The Single Parent's Scale	Never (0)	Rarely (1)	Sometimes (2)	Often (3)	Always (4)
1. To what extent does the therapist postulate the homeostatic maintainer (HM)?					
2. To what extent does the therapist intervene to transform the HM?					
3. To what extent does the therapist seek supportive opportunities for the children and parent (e.g., employment, training, health care)?					
4. To what extent do the therapist and parent recruit support (e.g., extended family, friends) to augment the parent's authority?					
5. To what extent does the therapist Join with the parent as an interim step?					
6. To what extent does the therapist conduct a search for areas of strength in the family?					
7. To what extent has the therapist established *sufficient* social supports for the parent such that there is a functional hierarchy?					
Total score:					

The Homeostatic Maintainer Searchlight	Never (0)	Rarely (1)	Sometimes (2)	Often (3)	Always (4)
1. To what extent does the therapist search within the family system to identify the HM?					
2. To what extent does the therapist perturb the system, noting who or what interactional pattern (the HM) activates to return the system to its status quo?					
3. To what extent does the therapist challenge and transform the HM?					
4. To what extent does the therapist reinforce the changes in the system; a new more functional status quo?					
Total score:					

Treatment Algorithms

Re: Chapter 8

IST Treatment of School Avoidance	Never (0)	Rarely (1)	Sometimes (2)	Often (3)	Always (4)
1. Therapist meets with parents to discuss the severity of the problem?					
2. Therapist facilitates parents meeting with school staff (teacher or counselor) to get daily or weekly feedback regarding attendance.					
3. The therapist advises parents (united) to take their youngster to school the next day. This may be repeated daily as necessary.					
Total score:					

IST Treatment of Failing Grades	Never (0)	Rarely (1)	Sometimes (2)	Often (3)	Always (4)
4. The therapist advises parental oversight of schoolwork; each parent chooses which topics to help their child with. Oversight should be nightly.					
5. The therapist advises parents and teachers to arrange performance feedback; meet every two weeks to review progress.					
6. Therapist advises parents to reward youngster if grades have improved at next marking period.					
7. To what extent does the therapist use the family therapy techniques? (Joining, Intensity, Enactments, Unbalancing, etc.)					
Total score:					

IST Treatment of Conduct Disorder	Never (0)	Rarely (1)	Sometimes (2)	Often (3)	Always (4)
1. To what extent does the therapist, with the team and family, determine the treatment goals using the Clinical Scorecard?					
2. To what extent does the therapist perturb the system?					
3. To what extent does the therapist identify the HM, the person who activates to rescue their child?					
4. To what extent does the therapist use family therapy techniques? A. For Joining? B. For Intensity? C. For Enactments? D. For Unbalancing?					
5. To what extent does the therapist create an Enactment between the parents to agree on a consequence and confront their young person?					
6. To what extent does the therapist utilize the Triangulation Scale or the Single Parent's Scale to determine readiness for discharge?					
7. To what extent does the therapist arrange for resources in the community to support the young person and their family when they are discharged?					
Total score:					

Re: Chapter 6

IST Treatment of Anorexia Nervosa (every clinical session)	Never (0)	Rarely (1)	Sometimes (2)	Often (3)	Always (4)
1. To what extent does the therapist create an organized system of care?					
2. To what extent does the therapist use the interactional patterns of the psychosomatic family?					
3. To what extent does the therapist address the isomorphic pattern of triangulation?					
4. To what extent does the therapist facilitate the parents working as a unit?					
5. To what extent does the therapist use the techniques of Intensity, Joining, Enactment, and Unbalancing?					
6. To what extent does the therapist initiate the therapy with either the lunch session or bed-rest protocol?					
7. To what extent does the therapist strengthen the parental unit during the bed-rest protocol or lunch session?					
8. To what extent does the therapist facilitate the family's tracking of the progress of weight gain?					
9. To what extent does the therapist help the family consult with the pediatrician or family doctor to monitor the patient's physical health?					
Total score:					

RE: Chapter 6

Tools On nzeatingdisorderspecialists.co.nz

Weight Gain Over Time

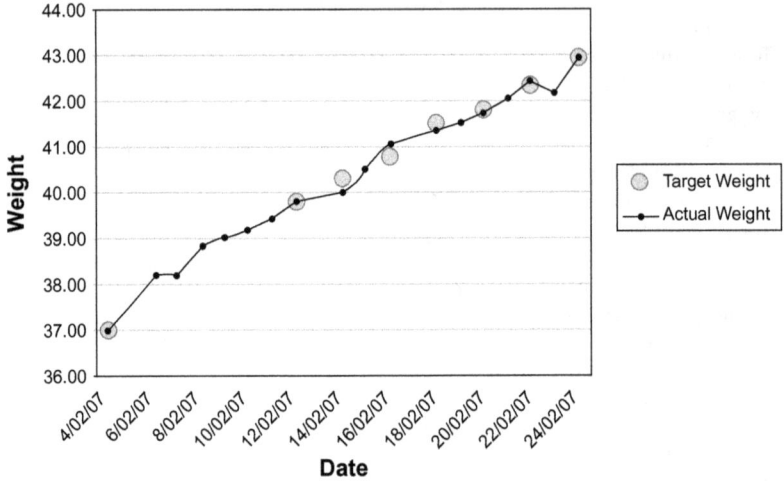

Weight Gain Personal Progress Guide (Example of Turning the Curve): Weight Gain Graph

New Zealand
Eating Disorder Specialists

This personal progress guide is for record purposes only. The figures noted are based on a patient record but not indicative of ideal calorie intake or actual weight. We suggest you consult a licenced professional for a controlled dietary plan.

For each day please record your calorie intake and actual weight. The corresponding charts will show your progress.

Enter your initial weight [83.1] pounds
Enter your target weight after 4 weeks [96.0] pounds

Actual vs Target Weight over Time

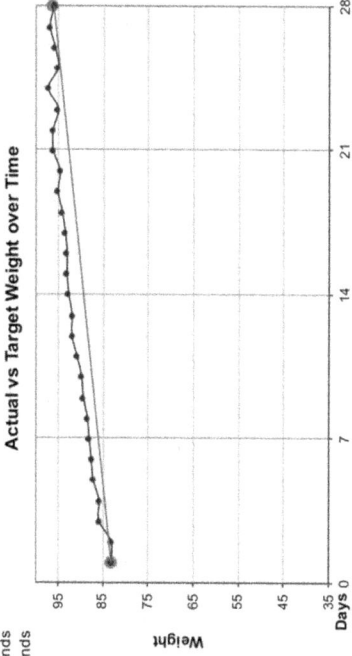

— Target Weight   —•— Actual Weight   —— Linear (Target Weight)

Daily Calorie Intake

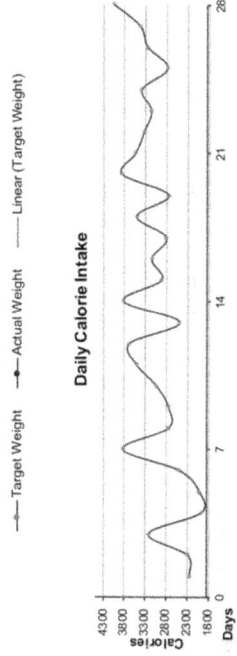

Week	Day	Calorie Intake	Actual Weight
1	1	2245	83.1
	2	2295	83.1
	3	3227	85.8
	4	1990	85.8
	5	2018	87.1
	6	2500	87.5
	7	3844	88.0
2	8	2757	88.4
	9	2757	89.3
	10	3045	89.7
	11	3521	90.8
	12	3675	91.9
	13	2493	91.9
	14	3834	92.6
3	15	2929	93.0
	16	3162	93.0
	17	2814	93.4
	18	3521	94.1
	19	2767	95.0
	20	3867	94.6
	21	3538	96.1
4	22	3340	96.1
	23	3170	95.0
	24	3395	97.2
	25	2790	95.0
	26	3263	95.7
	27	3438	96.8
	28	4043	95.9

Bulimia Nervosa and Compulsive Overeating Worksheet

Maria's weight gain personal progress guide. Maria's data applied to a computer tool for recording calorie intake, actual weight, and target weight, with graphs generated by the tool.

New Zealand
Eating Disorder Specialists

Week	Time and date mm/dd/yy 00:00	Incident or procrastination	Desire for bingeing/purging	Outcome Y/N	Conflict Score Did you address the conflict? Y = 0 N = 1
Example entry	*4/11/25 9:45*	*Please take notes here. The cell will expand and words wrap to provide more room as you type. To insert a new row (e.g., to add multiple entries per week): Click a cell in the row immediately below where you want the new row. For example, to insert a new row above Week 5, click a cell in row Week 5. Then, in the Insert menu, click Rows.*	*Please type only one of "bingeing" or "purging" in each cell below*	*Please note the cell will calculate every Y or N marked*	*0*
1					
2					
3					
4					
5					
6					
7					
8					
9					
10					

Your Dashboard	Incidence of bingeing	0	Incidence of N	0
Results at a Glance	Incidence of purging	0	Incidence of Y	0

Conflict Score total: 0

New Zealand Eating Disorders Bed-Rest Protocol for Your Child and Family

The bulimia nervosa and compulsive overeating worksheet—a spreadsheet for recording triggers to BN/COE.

This is a protocol that has been utilized many times to help eating disorder sufferers and their families get control of the self-starvation of anorexia nervosa. It is important to understand that this is done in conjunction with the patient's primary care physician. The primary care physician needs to see the patient weekly during the first crucial period. It is the primary care physician who determines whether medical hospitalization is necessary.

1	2	3	4	5
never	rarely	sometimes	often	always

It is an essential ingredient that the patient's weight needs to increase a certain amount, usually one pound every two or three days. There needs to be a precise scale that allows the parents to measure in ounces. She should wake up, go to the bathroom, then be weighed in the same clothes each time, such as a bathrobe.

1	2	3	4	5
never	rarely	sometimes	often	always

Should the patient not reach her weight gain target, e.g., one pound, she needs to have complete bed rest except for meals and toileting until she has regained the weight or achieved the target.

1	2	3	4	5
never	rarely	sometimes	often	always

While on bed rest, there is no TV or reading (there can be discussions with family members) while in bed. She should spend the time thinking about her life and dreams for the future.

1	2	3	4	5
never	rarely	sometimes	often	always

Ideally, both parents should be there to enforce the bed-rest protocol. When that's not possible, the parents can designate others (usually family members) to keep an eye on the patient and enforce the bed-rest protocol.

1	2	3	4	5
never	rarely	sometimes	often	always

Monitor attempts to contravene the protocol, e.g., putting stones in the bathrobe or drinking excessive amounts of water before being weighed.

1	2	3	4	5
never	rarely	sometimes	often	always

It is essential that both parents agree and support the protocol. If that is not the case, your family therapist must be contacted for an urgent consultation. This unity is crucial to the success of this approach.

1	2	3	4	5
never	rarely	sometimes	often	always

Utilize the weight gain and caloric intake protocol from the Tools for Change section, http://nzeatingdisorderspecialists.co.nz.

1	2	3	4	5
never	rarely	sometimes	often	always

Be sure that you understand the number of calories the patient must take in, usually between 2000 and 3000 per day. There can be nutritional supplements; caloric foods like thickshakes are to be encouraged.

1	2	3	4	5
never	rarely	sometimes	often	always

The patient should be encouraged to eat many times a day to avoid a bloated sensation.

1	2	3	4	5
never	rarely	sometimes	often	always

There should be collaboration between the family, your family therapist, and your child's primary care physician. We must all work together and be on the same page. If there are any questions or concerns, please contact your family therapist immediately.

1	2	3	4	5
never	rarely	sometimes	often	always

Re: Chapter 3 and 8

Alphabet of Skills Worksheet (from Minuchin and Fishman (1981), *Family Therapy Techniques*, Harvard University Press)

For each question, the sentence starts with "To what extent does the therapist..."

Educating the family	Never (0)	Rarely (1)	Sometimes (2)	Often (3)	Always (4)
1. ...provide useful information to help the family system change?					
2. ...give an interpretation, which is practical information, "if you work as a team, your child will be better behaved"?					
3. ...support the position of a member who is advocating positive change?					
4. ...provide a different, more practical definition of the problem?					
5. ...add valuable information toward positive change?					
6. ...bring others in to expand the family's options?					
Total score:					

Search for strength	Never (0)	Rarely (1)	Sometimes (2)	Often (3)	Always (4)
1. ...challenge the family's limited definition of a member's abilities?					
2. ...Unbalance the system, siding with the family member who is being strengthened?					
3. ...challenge the family to encourage their member to "stretch" and grow?					
4. ...support the family to re-contextualize, accessing new resources to enhance their family member's growth?					
Total score:					

Boundary making	Never (0)	Rarely (1)	Sometimes (2)	Often (3)	Always (4)
1. ...demonstrate the three types of boundary making?					
A. *As producer*: Introducing the concept of boundaries into the family system?					
B. *As director*: The therapist intervenes to facilitate the family in creating boundaries? e.g., "You shouldn't speak for your child."					
C. *As participant*: The therapist actively creates a boundary within the system? e.g., with changing seats					
2. ...demonstrate the appropriateness of boundaries within the family, against the developmental stages of the children?					
3. ...demonstrate boundary making as a cognitive construct?					
4. ...demonstrate boundary making as a time construct? e.g., the therapist intervenes to let people have more time to speak and make their point					
Total score:					

Joining	Never (0)	Rarely (1)	Sometimes (2)	Often (3)	Always (4)
1. ...demonstrate leadership in the session?					
2. ...demonstrate confirmation of all family members?					
3. ...demonstrate the ability to probe and question the family?					
4. ...demonstrate the capacity to give hope?					
5. To what extent is the therapist consistently non-judgmental?					
6. ...demonstrate tracking of the ongoing process?					
7. ...accommodate to the family rules initially?					
8. ...seek to find commonality with the family members?					
9. ...demonstrate the ability to be both inside and outside the family system?					
Total score:					

Intensity	Never (0)	Rarely (1)	Sometimes (2)	Often (3)	Always (4)
1. ...create Intensity by introducing dire consequences?					
2. ...use the Intensity of repetition?					
3. ...focus on the same issue for a longer period until there is change?					
4. ...resist the family's pressure to change the subject?					
5. ...demonstrate isomorphic interventions to increase Intensity? e.g., "When you and your husband don't get along, both of your boys behave in the same manner."					
6. ...demonstrate the ability to surpass the level of discomfort within the family such that different sequences emerge?					
7. ...tolerate the family's discomfort during the reframing process?					
8. ...demonstrate immovability when necessary?					
9. ...create Intensity by resisting family patterns?					
Total score:					

Enactment	Never (0)	Rarely (1)	Sometimes (2)	Often (3)	Always (4)
1. ...demonstrate ability at isolating sequences within the family that can be enacted?					
2. ...demonstrate ability to decentralize herself/himself?					
3. ...demonstrate the ability to allow family members to enact the sequence?					
4. ...demonstrate working toward the point of resolution?					
5. ...demonstrate the ability to continue the Enactment for a long period of time, often with repetition?					
6. ...demonstrate the ability to introduce alternatives as the Enactment is proceeding?					
7. ...demonstrate the ability to use Enactment to spread the problem from the identified person to that of the family sequences?					
8. ...frame sequences to be re-enacted?					
9. ...reinforce the change that has occurred?					
10. ...balloon small moments in the family session? e.g., "You smile when you discipline your child."					
11. ...resist the family's pressure to be central during Enactments?					
Total score:					

Complementarity	Never (0)	Rarely (1)	Sometimes (2)	Often (3)	Always (4)
1. …demonstrate the ability to intervene on the Complementarity of the interactions between family members, e.g., "Every time your alcoholic son runs out of wine, you buy it for him"?					
2. …demonstrate the ability to challenge the fixed ideas of a family by introducing the reciprocity of the behavior, e.g. "Perhaps you should see if your son will drink less if you supply less liquor"?					
3. …introduce a broader lens to the problem, utilizing the circularity of processes, e.g., "You're depressed, who's depressing you"?					
4. To what extent is the therapist able to punctuate the sessions to emphasize Complementarity, e.g., intervene to say, "When your daughter runs away and returns, you take her shopping, no wonder she continues to run away, you are rewarding her"?					
Total score:					

Unbalancing	Never (0)	Rarely (1)	Sometimes (2)	Often (3)	Always (4)
1. ...challenge the hierarchical pattern, often embedded in the family rules?					
2. ...side with one family member over another?					
3. ...track the interactional patterns within the family as they begin to change?					
4. ...support the family unit and confirm the individuals within the context of Unbalancing?					
5. ...resist the pull of the dominant family member?					
6. ...resist the pull of the neediest family member?					
7. ...maintain the Unbalancing until new patterns emerge?					
Total score:					

Re: Chapter 7

Windsor House Economic Assessment and Intervention Tool (used by Community Resource Specialist)

Workforce skills, educational attainment and labor force participation?

NAME_____DATE_____

---

1   2   3   4   5
low   high
Housing condition and location??
DATE_____

1   2   3   4   5
low   high
Participation in or knowledge of key institutions (family centers, religious institutions organised recreation) that reinforce social relationship and patterns of institutional consistency?
DATE_____

1   2   3   4   5
low   high
Access to reliable and quality child care and schooling?
DATE_____
CHILD'S NAME AND AGE _____
                        _____
                        _____

1   2   3   4   5
Low   high
Household budgeting, credit counselling and development of saving incentives and goals?
DATE_____

---

1   2   3   4   5
Low   high

Reflection Tool (for Supervisee)

Clinical Outcomes: Clinician Reflection Tool

Patient/Family	Problem	Outcome	1 Year Follow-Up	Lessons Learned

Consumer Feedback Evaluation Tool (The World's Shortest)

Chapter 5

Did we treat you well?
1   2   3   4   5
Did we help you with your problem?
1   2   3   4   5
Why did you rate us this way?

How can we do better?

Clinician's Mastery Report

Re: Chapter 8

Using a treatment protocol for conditions, that is, AN, School Avoidance, Failing Grades (you may, of course, use additional ones), measure episodes of care/patient from start to completion. Measure and reflect on clinical skills for each episode of care. Set targets and adjust as required. Turning the Curve shows the outcome of the case by looking at the slope of the curve. Composite scores are derived from the total number of episodes of care.

Dates (start/ completion)	Treatment protocols (measure with each episode of care)	Composite Score	% Targets Met	Outcome Turning the Curve slope (measurements over time)
	IST Treatment of AN (with each episode of care)			
	IST Treatment of School Avoidance (with each episode of care)			
	IST Treatment of Conduct Disorder (with each episode of care)			
	IST Treatment of Failing Grades (with each episode of care)			
	Homeostatic Maintainer Searchlight (with each episode of care)			
	IST Triangulation Scale (with each episode of care)			
	IST Single Parent Scale (with each episode of care)			

Dates (start/ completion)	Treatment protocols (measure with each episode of care)	Composite Score	% Targets Met	Outcome Turning the Curve slope (measurements over time)
	Alphabet of Skills Worksheet (measure with each episode of care) Joining Boundary Making Unbalancing Complementarity Enactment Intensity Search for strength Educating family			

IST-RBA Planning and Outcome Tracking

Re: Chapters 3, 4, and 5: IST Clinical Scorecard Worksheet

	Objectives/goals	Plans	Measures	Targets	HM/barriers
1					
2					
3					
...					

Targeting Tool

Date	Treatment plans	Measurements	Targets--% change over X period of time	Targets met

A Review of Accountable, Measurable Supervisory Schema

Re: Chapter 8

- Tracking the therapist's Use of Self-based on Alphabet of Skills Worksheet (likert scales).
- Tracking performance during a course of therapy using the Clinical Score Card (CSC). The clinician/team and the supervisor focus on the "Targets" column of the CSC to determine if the targets have been met.
- Tracking the episodes of therapy using the Turning the Curve Tool provides the measurements to determine whether the episode of therapy was successful; may also be used with episode composites.
- Tracking the use of the Triangulation Scale; tracking the therapist's scores on the treatment algorithms, the Homeostatic Maintainer Searchlight and the Single Parent Scale.
- The Clinician's Mastery Report registers performance measurements for the training clinician and the supervisor. Clinician's reflection is required for mastery.

REFERENCES

Attride-Stirling, J., Davis, H., Stevenless, G., Sclare, I., & Day, C. (2001). "Someone to talk to who'll listen": Addressing the psychosocial needs of children and families. *Journal of Community & Applied Social Psychology, 11*(3) 179–191. https://doi.org/10.1002/casp.613

Avila, A., Distelberg, B., Estrada, A., Samman, S., Borieux, M., Yektafar, G., & Moline, M. (2016). Developing dyadic evaluation for supervision: An exploratory factor analysis. *Contemporary Family Therapy, 38*, 284–294. https://doi.org/10.1007/s10591-016-9388-4

Avildsen, J. G. (1989). *Lean on me* [Film]. Warner Bros.

Banovcinova, A., Levicka, J., & Veres, M. (2014, May 15). The impact of poverty on the family system functioning. *Procedia: Social and Behavioral Sciences. 132*, 148–153. https://doi.org/10.1016/j.sbspro.2014.04.291

Bateson, G. (1972). *Steps to an ecology of mind.* University of Chicago Press.

Bateson, G. (2002). *Mind and nature: A necessary unity.* Hampton Press. (Original work published 1979).

Berwick, D. M. (2007). *Eating soup with a fork* [Video]. Institute for Health Care Improvement. http://www.ihi.org/resources/Pages/AudioandVideo/Don-Berwick-Forum-Keynotes.aspx

Berwick, D. M. (2019). *Quality, mercy and the moral determinants of health* [Video]. Institute for Healthcare Improvement. http://www.ihi.org/resources/Pages/AudioandVideo/Don-Berwick-Forum-Keynotes.aspx

Berwick, D. M. (2020). The moral determinants of health. *JAMA, 324*(3), 225–226. https://doi.org/10.1001/jama.202011129

Berwick, D. M., Godfrey, A. B., & Roessner, J. (1991). *Curing health care: New strategies for quality improvement.* Jossey-Bass.

Berwick, D. M., James, B., & Coye, M. J. (2003). Connections between quality measurement and improvement, *Medical Care, 41*(1 Suppl), I30–8. https://doi.org/10.1097/00005650-200301001-00004

Blanchard, K. H. (2003). *The one minute manager.* Morrow.

Bögels, S., Hoogstad, B., van Dun, L., de Schutter, S., & Restifo, K. (2008). Mindfulness training for adolescents with externalizing disorders and their parents. *Behavioural and Cognitive Psychotherapy, 36*(2), 193–209. https://doi.org/10.1017/S1352465808004190

Bond, M. (2014). *The power of others: Peer pressure, groupthink and how the people around us shape everything we do.* Oneworld.

Breslow, J. M. (2012, September 21). *By the numbers: Dropping out of high school.* NPR. http://www.pbs.org/wgbh/frontline/article/by-the-num bers-dropping-out-of-high-school/

Breunlin, D. C., Pinsof, W., Russell, W. P., & Lebow, J. (2011). Integrative problem-centered metaframeworks therapy: Core concepts and hypothesizing. *Family Process, 50,* 292–313. https://doi.org/10.1111/j. 1545-5300.2011.01362.x

Bringewatt, E. H., & Gershoff, E. T. (2010). Falling through the cracks: Gaps and barriers in the mental health system for America's disadvantaged children. *Children and Youth Services Review, 32*(10), 1291–1299. https:// doi.org/10.1016/j.childyouth.2010.04.021

Burns, B. J., Angold, A., Tweed, D., Stangl, D., Farmer, E. M., & Erkanli, A. (1995). Children's mental health service use across service sectors. *Health Affairs, 14*(3) 147–159.

Busch, R. (2011). *Contextualising a problematic relationship between narrative therapy and evidence-based psychotherapy evaluation in psychology* [Unpublished PhD thesis]. Massey University. http://hdl.handle.net/ 10179/2986

Carey, B. (2015, August 27). Many psychology findings not as strong as claimed, study says. *The New York Times.* https://www.nytimes.com/ 2015/08/28/science/many-social-science-findings-not-as-strong-as-claimed-study-says.html

Carr, A. (2014). The evidence base for family therapy and systemic interventions for child-focused problems" *Journal of Family Therapy*, 36(2), 107–157. https://doi.org/10.1111/1467-6427.12032

Chen, Y., Kelton, C. M., Jing, Y., Guo, J. J., Li, X., & Patel, N. C. (2008). Utilization, price, and spending trends for antidepressants in the US Medicaid Program. *Research in Social and Administrative Pharmacy*, 4(3), 244–257. https://doi.org/10.1016/j.sapharm.2007.06.019

Choudry, I. (2018, March 19). High school dropouts more likely to go to prison. *Spotlight*. https://slspotlight.com/opinion/2018/03/19/high-school-dropouts-more-likely-to-go-to-prison/

Claridge, J. A., & Fabian, T. C. (2005). History and development of evidence-based medicine. *World Journal of Surgery*, 29(5), 547–553.

Clayworth, P. (2012, June 20). Prisons: New Zealand's prisons. In *Te ara: The encyclopedia of New Zealand*. http://www.teara.govt.nz/en/prisons/page-1

Cochrane, A. L. (1972). *Effectiveness and efficiency: Random reflections on health services*. Nuffield Provincial Hospitals Trust.

Coid, J. (2003). Formulating strategies for the primary prevention of adult antisocial behaviour: "High risk" or "population" strategies? In D. Farrington & J. Coid (Eds.), *Early Prevention of Adult Antisocial Behaviour. Cambridge Studies in Criminology* (pp. 32–78). Cambridge University Press. doi:10.1017/CBO9780511489259.003

Cook, J. M., Biyanova, T., Elhai, J., Schnurr, P. P., & Coyne, J. C. (2010). What do psychotherapists really do in practice? An internet study of over 2,000 practitioners. *Psychotherapy: Theory, Research, Practice, Training*, 47(2), 260–267. https://doi.org/10.1037/a0019788

Cottrell, D., & Boston, P. (2002). Practitioner review: The effectiveness of systemic family therapy for children and adolescents. *Journal of Child Psychology and Psychiatry*, 43: 573–586. https://doi.org/10.1111/1469-7610.00047

Cross, T., Bazron, B., Dennis, K., & Isaacs, M. (1989). *Towards a culturally competent system of care: A monograph on effective services for minority children who are severely emotionally disturbed*. Georgetown University Child Development Center, CASSP Technical Assistance Center.

Cui, L., Hung, H. M., & Wang, S. J. (1999, September). Modification of sample size in group sequential clinical trials. *Biometrics*, 55(3), 853–857. https://doi.org/10.1111/j.0006-341x.1999.00853.x

Deloitte Access Economics. (2020, June). *Social and economic cost of eating disorders in the United States of America*. Report for the Strategic Training Initiative for the Prevention of Eating Disorders and the Academy for Eating Disorders. https://cdn1.sph.harvard.edu/wp-content/uploads/sites/1267/2020/06/Social-Economic-Cost-of-Eating-Disorders-in-US-5.pdf

Dickersin, K., Chan, S. S., Chalmers, T. C., Sacks, H. S., & Smith Jr., H. (1987). Publication bias and clinical trials. *Controlled Clinical Trials, 8*(4), 343–353.

Doerr, J. (2018). *Measure what matters*. Portfolio Penguin.

Edmonds, L. K., Williams, S., & Walsh, A. E. S. (2000). Trends in Maori mental health in Otago. *Australian & New Zealand Journal of Psychiatry, 34*(4), 677–683.

Edwards, B. (2015). *Breaking the vicious cycle: 5 family therapy interventions*. GoodTherapy. https://www.goodtherapy.org/blog/breaking-the-vicious-cycle-5-family-therapy-interventions-0106154

Every-Palmer, S., & Howick, J. (2014). How evidence-based medicine is failing due to biased trials and selective publication. *Journal of Evaluation in Clinical Practice, 20*(6), 908–914. https://doi.org/10.1111/jep.12147

Fanelli, D. (2009). How many scientists fabricate and falsify research? A systematic review and meta-analysis of survey data. *PLoS One, 4*(5), e5738. https://doi.org/10.1371/journal.pone.0005738

Fang, F. C., Steen R. G., & Casadevall, A. (2012). Misconduct accounts for the majority of retracted scientific publications. *Proceedings of the National Academy of Sciences of the United States of America, 109*(42), 17028–17033. https://doi.org/10.1073/pnas.1212247109

Fishman, H. C. (2004). *Enduring change in eating disorders: Interventions with long-term results*. Brunner-Routledge.

Fishman, H. C. (2017, December 10). Personal reflections on Salvador Minuchin. *IST*. https://intensivestructuraltherapy.com/2017/12/10/personal-reflections-on-salvador-minuchin/

Fishman, H. C., Scott, S., & Betof, N. (1977, August 1). A hall of mirrors: A structural approach to the problems of the mentally retarded. *Mental Retardation, 15*(4), 24.

Fishman, H. C., Andes, F., & Knowlton, R. (2001). Enhancing family therapy: The addition of a Community Resource Specialist. *Journal of Marital and Family Therapy, 27*(1), 111–116.

Flåm, A. M. (2016). Dialogical research in supervision: Practical guidelines from experienced supervisors in family therapy, child protection, and specialty mental health services. *Australian & New Zealand Journal of Family Therapy, 37*(3), 282–296. https://doi.org/10.1002/anzf.1158

Fowler, J. H., & Christakis, N. A. (2008, February). Dynamic spread of happiness in a large social network: Longitudinal analysis over 20 years in the Framingham Heart Study. *British Medical Journal, 337*(dec04_2), a2338. https://doi: 10.1136/bmj.a2338

Frank, G. (1984). The Boulder model: History, rationale and critique. *Professional Psychology: Research and Practice, 15*(3), 417–435. https://doi.org/10.1037/0735-7028.15.3.417

Freedman, D. H. (2010a, June 10). Wrong. *The New York Times.* https://www.nytimes.com/2010/06/11/books/excerpt-wrong.html

Freedman, D. H. (2010b, November). Lies, damned lies, and medical science. *The Atlantic.* https://www.theatlantic.com/magazine/archive/2010/11/lies-damned-lies-and-medical-science/308269/

Friedman, M. (2015). *Trying hard is not good enough: How to produce measurable improvements for customers and communities* (3rd ed.). CreateSpace.

Fugh-Berman, A., & Ahari, S. (2007). Following the scripS: How drug reps make friends and influence doctors (policy forum). *PLoS Medicine, 4*(4), e150. https://doi.org/10.1371/journal.pmed.0040150

Godlee, F. (2014). Evidence-based medicine: flawed system but still the best we've got. *BMJ, 348,* g440.

Goldacre, B. (2017, December 5). Evidence to House of Commons Sci Tech Select Committee on Research Integrity. *Bad Science.* www.badscience.net/2017/12/evidence-to-house-of-commons-sci-tech-select-committee-on-research-integrity/#more-3498

Gomory, T. (2013). The limits of evidence-based medicine and its application to mental health evidence-based practice: Part one. *Ethical Human Psychology and Psychiatry, 15*(1), 18–34.

Goodman, S. N. (1999). Toward evidence-based medical statistics. 1: The *p* value fallacy. *Annals of Internal Medicine, 130*(12), 995–1004.

Gratzer, W. (2013). Trouble at the lab. *The Economist, 302*(5911), 774–775. https://www.economist.com/briefing/2013/10/18/trouble-at-the-lab

Greenhalgh, T., Howick, J., & Maskrey, N. (2014). Evidence based medicine: A movement in crisis?. *BMJ* (Clinical research ed.), *348*, g3725. https://doi.org/10.1136/bmj.g3725

Haley, J. (1969). *The power tactics of jesus christ, and other essays* (1st ed.). Grossman.

Haley, J. (1976). *Problem-solving therapy*. Jossey-Bass.

Hamilton, C. (2016). What 'treatment as usual' costs in Australia. National Eating Disorders Association. https://www.nationaleatingdisorders.org/blog/what-treatment-usual-costs-australia

Harris, J. R. (2016). What do you consider the most interesting recent (scientific) news? What makes it important? *Edge.* https://www.edge.org/response-detail/26682

Harrison, M. E., McKay, M. M., & Bannon, W. M. (2004). Inner-city child mental health service use: The real question is why youth and families do not use services. *Community Mental Health Journal, 40*(2), 119–131. https://doi.org/10.1023/B:COMH.0000022732.80714.8b

He, T. (2013). Retraction of global scientific publications from 2001 to 2010. *Scientometrics, 96*(2), 555–561.

Heatherington, L., Messer, S. B., Angus, L., Strauman, T. J., Friedlander, M. L., & Kolden, G. G. (2012). The narrowing of theoretical orientations in clinical psychology doctoral training. *Clinical Psychology: Science and Practice, 19*(4), 364–374. https://doi.org/10.1111/cpsp.12012

Henggeler, S. W., & Sheidow, A. J. (2012). Empirically supported family-based treatments for conduct disorder and delinquency in adolescents. *Journal of Marital and Family Therapy, 38*(1), 30–58. https://doi.org/10.1111/j.1752-0606.2011.00244.x

Heres, S., Davis, J., Maino, K., Jetzinger, E., Kissling, W., & Leucht, S. (2006). Why olanzapine beats risperidone, risperidone beats quetiapine, and quetiapine beats olanzapine: An exploratory analysis of head-to-head comparison studies of second-generation antipsychotics. *American Journal of Psychiatry, 163*(2), 185–194. https://doi.org/10.1176/appi.ajp.163.2.185

Hodges, K., & Kim, C. (2000). Psychometric study of the Child and Adolescent Functional Assessment Scale: Prediction of contact with the law and poor school attendance. *Journal of Abnormal Child Psychology, 28*, 287–297. https://doi.org/10.1023/A:1005100521818

Hodgson, J. L., Johnson, L. N., Ketring, S. A., Wampler, R. S., & Lamson, A. L. (2005, January). Integrating research and clinical training in marriage and family therapy training programs. *Journal of Marital and Family Therapy, 31*(1), 75–88. https://doi.org/10.1111/j.1752-0606.2005.tb01544.x

Horton, R. (2015, April 11). Offline: What is medicine's 5 sigma? *Lancet, 385*(9976), 1380. https://www.thelancet.com/journals/lancet/article/PIIS0140-6736(15)60696-1/fulltext

Hutchings, J., Bywater, T., Daley, D., Gardner, F., Whitaker, C., Jones, K., Eames, C., & Edwards, R. T. (2007, March 31). Parenting intervention in Sure Start Services for children at risk of developing conduct disorder: Pragmatic randomized controlled trial. *BMJ, 334,* 678–684. https://doi.org/10.1136/bmj.39126.620799.55

Ilyas, S., & Moncrieff, J. (2012). Trends in prescriptions and costs of drugs for mental disorders in England, 1998–2010. *The British Journal of Psychiatry: The Journal of Mental Science, 200*(5), 393–398. https://doi.org/10.1192/bjp.bp.111.104257

Imber-Black, E. (2014). Eschewing certainties: The creation of family therapists in the 21st century. *Family Process, 53*(3), 371–379. https://doi.org10.1111/famp.12091

Insel, T. (2012, February 24). Spotlight on eating disorders. NIH, National Institute of Mental Health. https://www.nimh.nih.gov/about/directors/thomas-insel/blog/2012/spotlight-on-eating-disorders.shtml

Ioannidis, J. P. (2003). Genetic associations: False or true? *Trends in Molecular Medicine, 9*(4), 135–138.

Ioannidis, J. P. (2005). Why most published research findings are false. *PLoS Medicine, 2*(8), e124. https://doi.org/10.1371/journal.pmed.0020124

Ioannidis, J. P. (2020, July). Spin, bias, and clinical utility in systematic reviews of diagnostic studies. *Clinical Chemistry, 66*(7), 863–865. https://doi.org/10.1093/clinchem/hvaa114

Ioannidis, J. P., & Trikalinos, T. A. (2007). The appropriateness of asymmetry tests for publication bias in meta-analyses: A large survey. *Canadian Medical Association Journal, 176*(8), 1091–1096.

Ioannidis, J. P., Ntzani, E. E., Trikalinos, T. A., & Contopoulos-Ioannidis, D. G. (2001). Replication validity of genetic association studies. *Nature Genetics, 29*(3), 306.

Jørgensen, A. W., Hilden, J., & Gøtzsche, P. C. (2006). Cochrane reviews compared with industry supported meta-analyses and other meta-analyses of the same drugs: Systematic review. *BMJ* (Clinical research ed.), *333*(7572), 782. https://doi.org/10.1136/bmj.38973.444699.0B

Kamenetz, A. (2015, June 12). *From 'dropout crisis' to record high, dissecting the graduation rate.* NPR. https://www.npr.org/sections/ed/2015/06/12/411751159/the-story-behind-the-record-high-graduation-rate

Kantor, E. D., Rehm, C. D., Haas, J. S., Chan, A. T., & Giovannucci, E. L. (2015). Trends in prescription drug use among adults in the United States from 1999–2012. *JAMA, 314*(17), 1818–1831. https://doi.org/10.1001/jama.2015.13766

Karam, E. A., & Sprenkle, D. H. (2010, July). The research-informed clinician: A guide to training the next-generation MFT. *Journal of Marital and Family Therapy, 36*(3), 307–319. https://doi.org/10.1111/j.1752-0606.2009.00141.x. PMID: 20618578.

Karamat Ali, R., & Bachicha, D. L. (2012, April). Systemic supervision practices compared: A closer look at 'reflection' and 'self' in multisystemic therapy and family therapy supervision. *Clinical Child Psychology and Psychiatry, 17*(2), 192–207. https://doi.org/10.1177/1359104512442058

Kiresuk, T. J., & Sherman, R. E. (1968, December). Goal attainment scaling: A general method for evaluating comprehensive community mental health programs. *Community Mental Health Journal, 4*(6), 443–453. https://doi.org/10.1007/BF01530764

Koltz, R. L., Odegard, M. A., Feit, S. S., Provost, K., & Smith, T. (2012) Parallel process and isomorphism: A model for decision making in the supervisory triad. *The Family Journal, 20*(3), 233–238.

Kuhn, T. S. (1962). *The Structure of Scientific Revolutions.* University of Chicago Press.

Lam, B. (2015, September). A scientific look at bad science. *The Atlantic.* https://www.theatlantic.com/magazine/archive/2015/09/a-scientific-look-at-bad-science/399371/

Leeds City Council. (2015). *Leeds children and young people's plan for 2015–19. From good to great.* http://democracy.leeds.gov.uk/documents/s132827/94%20App%203%20cyppfinaleb2406.pdf

Leichsenring, F., & Steinert, C. (2017). Is cognitive behavioral therapy the gold standard for psychotherapy?: The need for plurality in treatment and research. *JAMA, 318*(14), 1323–1324. https://doi.org/10.1001/jama. 2017.13737

Leichsenring, F., Steinert, C., & Ioannidis, J. P. (2019). Toward a paradigm shift in treatment and research of mental disorders. *Psychological Medicine*, 1–7. https://doi.org/10.1017/S0033291719002265

Levin, H. M., & Rouse, C. E. (2012, January 25). The true cost of high school dropouts. *The New York Times*. https://www.nytimes.com/2012/01/26/opinion/the-true-cost-of-high-school-dropouts.html

Lévi-Strauss, C. (1962). *The savage mind*. University of Chicago Press.

Lincoln, T., Wilhelm, K., & Nestoriuc, Y. (2007, December). Effectiveness of psychoeducation for relapse, symptoms, knowledge, adherence and functioning in psychotic disorders: A meta-analysis. *Schizophrenia Research, 96*(1–3), 232–245.

Littell, J. H., Popa, M., & Forsythe, B. (2005, July 20). Multisystemic therapy for social, emotional, and behavioral problems in youth aged 10–17. *The Cochrane Database of Systematic Reviews, 3*, CD004797. https://doi.org/10.1002/14651858.CD004797.pub3

MacKay, G., Somerville, W., & Lundie, J. (1996). Reflections on goal attainment scaling (GAS): Cautionary notes and proposals for development. *Educational Research, 38*(2), 161–172. https://doi.org/10.1080/0013188960380204

Meadows, D. H. (2008). *Thinking in systems: A primer*. Chelsea Green Publishing.

Millenson, M. L. (2003). *Getting doctors to say yes to drugs: The cost and quality of impact of drug company marketing to physicians*. Blue Cross Blue Shield Association. Accessed October 9, 2018. http://www.bcbs.com/betterknowledge/cost/ getting-doctors-to-say-yes.html

Mills, C. F., Tobias, M., & Baker, M. (2002). A re-appraisal of the burden of infectious disease in New Zealand: Aggregate estimates of morbidity and mortality. *Journal of the New Zealand Medical Association, 115*(1155), 254–257.

Minuchin, S. (1974). *Families and family therapy*. Harvard University Press.

Minuchin, S. (1998). Where is the family in narrative family therapy. *The Journal of Marriage and Family Therapy, 24*(4), 397–403.

Minuchin, S., & Fishman, H. C. (1979). The psychosomatic family in child psychiatry. *Journal of the American Academy of Child Psychiatry, 18*(1), 76–90.

Minuchin, S., & Fishman, H. C. (1981). *Family therapy techniques*. Harvard University Press.

Minuchin, S., Montalvo, B., Guerney, Jr., B. G., Rosman, B. L., & Schumer, F. (1967). *Families of the slums: An exploration of their structure and treatment*. Basic Books.

Minuchin, S., Rosman, B. L., & Baker, L. (1978). *Psychosomatic families: Anorexia nervosa in context*. Harvard University Press.

Morgan, A. (2000). *What is narrative therapy? An easy to read introduction*. Dulwich Centre Publications.

Morgan, M. M., & Sprenkle, D. H. (2007, January). Toward a common-factors approach to supervision. *Journal of Marital and Family Therapy, 33*(1), 1–17.

Narayan, D., Chalmers, R., Shah, M. K., & Petesch, P. (2000a). *Voices of the poor: Crying out for change*. Oxford University Press for the World Bank.

Narayan, D., Patel, R. & World Bank. (2000b). *Voices of the poor: Can anyone hear us?* Oxford University Press.

Newton, I. (1675). Letter to Robert Hooke. Retrieved from https://digitallibrary.hsp.org/index.php/Detail/objects/9792#

NHS. (n.d.) *Treatment: Anorexia nervosa*. https://www.nhs.uk/conditions/anorexia/treatment/

Northey Jr., W. F. (2002). Characteristics and clinical practices of marriage and family therapists: A national survey. *Journal of Marital and Family Therapy, 28*(4), 487–494.

NZ Drug Foundation. (2013, February). The cost of our convictions. *Matters of Substance, 24*(1). https://www.drugfoundation.org.nz/matters-of-substance/february-2013/cost-of-our-convictions/

Open Science Collaboration. (2015). Psychology. Estimating the reproducibility of psychological science. *Science, 349*(6251), aac4716. https://doi.org/10.1126/science.aac4716

PBS NewsHour. (2014, March 3). *Low income students combat stress with mindfulness*. https://www.pbs.org/video/low-income-students-combat-stress-with-mindfulness-1401142061/

Perlis, R. H., Perlis, C. S., Wu, Y., Hwang, C., Joseph, M., & Nierenberg, A. A. (2005). Industry sponsorship and financial conflict of interest in the reporting of clinical trials in psychiatry. *American Journal of Psychiatry, 162*(10), 1957–1960. https://doi.org/10.1176/appi.ajp.162.10.1957

Perou, R., Bitsko, R. H., Blumberg, S. J., Pastor, P., Ghandour, R. M., Gfroerer, J. C., Hedden, S. L., Crosby, A. E., Visser, S. N., Schieve, L. A., Parks, S. E., Hall, J. E., Brody, D., Simile, C. M., Thompson, W. W., Baio, J., Avenevoli, S., Kogan, M. D., Huang, L. N., & Centers for Disease Control and Prevention (CDC). (2013). Mental health surveillance among children--United States, 2005–2011. *MMWR supplements*, 62(2), 1–35.

Putnam, R. D. (2015). *Our kids: The American dream in crisis*. Simon & Schuster.

PwC. (2015). *The costs of eating disorders: Social, health, and economic impacts*. Beat. https://www.beateatingdisorders.org.uk/uploads/documents/2017/10/the-costs-of-eating-disorders-final-original.pdf

Raimy, V. C. (Ed.). (1950). *Training in clinical psychology*. Prentice-Hall.

Rigazio-DiGilio, S. A. (2014). Supervising couple and family therapy practitioners. In C. E. Watkins and D. Milne (Eds.), *The Wiley International Handbook of Clinical Supervision* (pp. 622–647). Wiley-Blackwell.

Ringel, J. S., & Sturm, R. (2001). National estimates of mental health utilization and expenditures for children in 1998. *The Journal of Behavioral Health Services and Research, 28*(3), 319–333. https://doi.org/10.1007/BF02287247

Rogers, A. (2017, November 5). Star neuroscientist Tom Insel leaves the Google-spawned Verily for ... a startup? *Wired*. https://www.wired.com/2017/05/star-neuroscientist-tom-insel-leaves-google-spawned-verily-startup/

Rynes, K. N., Rohrbaugh, M. J., Lebensohn-Chialvo, F., & Shoham, V. (2014). Parallel demand-withdraw processes in family therapy for adolescent drug abuse. *Psychology of addictive behaviors: Journal of the Society of Psychologists in Addictive Behaviors, 28*(2), 420–430. https://doi.org/10.1037/a0031812

Sackett, D. L. (1997). Evidence-based medicine. *Seminars in Perinatology, 21*(1), 3–5. https://doi.org/10.1016/s0146-0005(97)80013-4

Sandplay Therapists of America. (n.d.) *What is sandplay therapy*. https://www.sandplay.org/about-sandplay/what-is-sandplay

Schoenwald, S. K., & Hoagwood, K. (2001). Effectiveness, transportability, and dissemination of interventions: What matters when? *Psychiatric Services, 52*(9), 1190–1197.

Schoenwald, S. K., Sheidow, A. J., & Chapman, J. E. (2009). Clinical supervision in treatment transporS: Effects on adherence and outcomes. *Journal of Consulting and Clinical Psychology, 77*(3), 410–421. https://doi.org/10.1037/a0013788

Schorr, L. B. (2016, January 8). Reconsidering evidence: What it means and how we use it. *Stanford Social Innovation Review.* https://ssir.org/articles/entry/reconsidering_evidence_what_it_means_and_how_we_use_it

Schorr, L. B., & Farrow, F. (2011, July). *Expanding the evidence universe: Doing better by knowing more.* Center for the Study of Social Policy. pathways.nccp.org/assets/pdf/SchorrFarrow2011.pdf

Schulz, K. F., & Grimes, D. A. (2005, April 9–15). Sample size calculations in randomised trials: Mandatory and mystical. *Lancet, 365*(9467), 1348–1353. https://doi.org/10.1016/S0140-6736(05)61034-3

Sen, A. K. (2000). *Social exclusion: Concept, application, and scrutiny.* Asian Development Bank.

Sexton, T. L., Kinser, J. C., & Hanes, C. W. (2008). Beyond a single standard: Levels of evidence approach for evaluating marriage and family therapy research and practice. *Journal of Family Therapy, 30*(4), 386–398. https//doi.org/10.1111/j.1467-6427.2008.00444.x

Signal, L., Martin, J., Cram, F., & Robson, B. (2008). *The health equity assessment tool: A user's guide.* Ministry of Health. https://www.health.govt.nz/publication/health-equity-assessment-tool-users-guide

Simmons, D., & Voyle, J. A. (2003). Reaching hard-to-reach, high-risk populations: Piloting a health promotion and diabetes disease prevention programme on an urban marae in New Zealand. *Health Promotion International, 18*(1), 41–50.

Simmons, J. P., Nelson, L. D., & Simonsohn, U. (2011). False-positive psychology: Undisclosed flexibility in data collection and analysis allows presenting anything as significant. *Psychological Science, 22*(11), 1359–1366. https://doi.org/10.1177/0956797611417632

Singh, N. N., Lancioni, G. E., Singh Joy, S. D., Winton, A. S., Sabaawi, M., Wahler, R. G., & Singh, J. (2007). Adolescents with conduct disorder can be mindful of their aggressive behavior. *Journal of Emotional and Behavioral Disorders, 15*(1), 56–63. https://doi.org/10.1177/1063426607015001060

Smith, A. R., Zuromski, K. L., & Dodd, D. R. (2018). Eating disorders and suicidality: What we know, what we don't know, and suggestions for future research. *Current Opinion in Psychology, 22*, 63–67. https://doi.org/10.1016/j.copsyc.2017.08.023

Snelle, M. (2015, September 25). From care to incarceration: The relationship between adverse childhood experience and dysfunctionality in later life. *Independent.* https://www.independent.co.uk/life-style/health-and-families/features/care-incarceration-relationship-between-adverse-childhood-experience-and-dysfunctionality-later-life-10409737.html

Strein, W., Hoagwood, K., & Cohn, A. (2003). School psychology: A public health perspective: I. Prevention, populations, and systems change. *Journal of School Psychology, 41*(1), 23–38. doi: 10.1016/S0022-4405(02)00142-5

Stricker, G. (2006). The local clinical scientist, evidence-based practice, and personality assessment. *Journal of Personality Assessment, 86*(1), 4–9. https://doi.org/10.1207/s15327752jpa8601_02

Stroul, B., Blau, G., & Friedman, R. (2010). *Updating the system of care concept and philosophy.* Georgetown University Center for Child and Human Development, National Technical Assistance Center for Children's Mental Health.

Sumerel, M. B. (1994). Parallel process in supervision. *ERIC Digest,* April. https://eric.ed.gov/?id=ED372347

Synergos Institute. (n.d.). *Social connectedness program.* https://bettercarenetwork.org/sites/default/files/Social%20Connectedness%20Programme.pdf

TEDx. (2014, February 28). *Molly McGrath Tierney: Re-thinking foster care* [Video]. YouTube. https://www.youtube.com/watch?v=c15hy8dXSps

Thaler, R. H., & Sunstein, C. R. (2008). *Nudge: Improving decisions about health, wealth, and happiness.* Yale University Press.

The Annie E. Casey Foundation. (n.d.). *About Us.* https://aecf.org/about/

Todd, T. C., & Storm, C. L. (2014). *The complete systemic supervisor: Context, philosophy, and pragmatics* (2nd ed.). Wiley-Blackwell.

Tolstoy, L. (2004). *Anna Karenina.* Translated by R. Pevear & L. Volokhonsky. Penguin. (Original work published 1877).

Turner, E. H., Matthews, A. M., Linardatos, E., Tell, R. A., and Rosenthal, R. (2008). Selective publication of antidepressant trials and its influence on apparent efficacy. *New England Journal of Medicine, 358*(3), 252–260.

UNICEF. (2001). *A league table of teenage births in rich nations.* Innocenti Report Card no. 3.

United Press International News Track. (2004). *New Zealand teen suicide the highest.* http://www.washtimes.com/upi-breaking/20040607-110646-8431r.htm

Vallas, R., & Boteach, M. (2014, September 17). *The top 10 solutions to cut poverty and grow the middle class.* Center for American Progress. https://www.americanprogress.org/issues/poverty/news/2014/0 9/17/97287/the-top-10-solutions-to-cut-poverty-and-grow-the-midd le-class/

VC News Daily. (n.d.). *Wealthiest VCs.* https://vcnewsdaily.com/Wealthiest _VCs.php

Wallace, K., & Cooper, M. (2015, March). Development of supervision personalisation forms: A qualitative study of the dimensions along which supervisors' practices vary. *Counselling and Psychotherapy Research, 15*(1), 31–40. https://doi.org/10.1002/capr.12001

Watkins, C. E. Jr. (2011) Does Psychotherapy Supervision Contribute to Patient Outcomes? Considering Thirty Years of Research, *The Clinical Supervisor, 30*(2), 235–256. https://doi.org/10.1080/0732522 3.2011.619417

Weisz, J. R., & Kazdin, A. E. (2010). *Evidence-based psychotherapies for children and adolescents.* Guilford Press.

Weltzin, T. E., Weisensel, N., Franczyk, D., Burnett, K., Klitz, C., & Bean, P. (2005, June). Eating disorders in men: Update. *Journal of Men's Health and Gender, 2*(2), 186–193. https://doi.org/10.1016/j.jmhg.2005.04.008

Wetzel, N. A., & Winawer, H. (2011). Social justice in clinical practice: Family consultations with adolescents in urban schools: Part 1. *New Jersey Psychologist, 61*(4), 40–42.

Whittington, C. J., Kendall, T., Fonagy, P., Cottrell, D., Cotgrove, A., and Boddington, F. (2004). Selective serotonin reuptake inhibitors in childhood depression: Systematic review of published versus unpublished data. *The Lancet, 363*(9418): 1341–1345.

Xue, Y., Leventhal, T., Brooks-Gunn, J., & Earls, F. J. (2005). Neighborhood residence and mental health problems of 5- to 11-year-olds. *Archives of General Psychiatry*, 62(5): 554–563. https://doi.org/10.1001/archpsyc. 62.5.554

Zak, P. (2013, July 4). *Measurement myopia*. Drucker Institute. https://www. drucker.institute/thedx/measurement-myopia/

INDEX

For Product Safety Concerns and Information please contact our EU
representative GPSR@taylorandfrancis.com
Taylor & Francis Verlag GmbH, Kaufingerstraße 24, 80331 München, Germany